PocketRadiologist™
Interventional
Top 100 Procedures

PocketRadiologist™
Interventional
Top 100 Procedures

Peter Rogers MD
Interventional Radiologist and Neuroradiologist
Hines Veterans Hospital
Hines, Illinois

Clinical Instructor, Interventional Radiology and Neuroradiology
Loyola University, Residency Program
Maywood, Illinois

Anne Roberts MD
Professor of Radiology
University of California, San Diego
Thornton Hospital
La Jolla, California

Peter Schloesser MD
Assistant Professor Interventional Neuroradiology
University of Utah School of Medicine
Salt Lake City, Utah

Wade Wong DO FACR
Professor of Radiology
University of California, San Diego
San Diego, California

With contribution by: *Michael Preece*

With 200 drawings and radiographic images

Drawings: *Lane R Bennion MS*
              Richard Coombs MS
              James A Cooper MD
Image Editing: *Ming Q Huang MD*
              Danielle Morris
              Melissa Petersen

AMIRSYS™

W. B. SAUNDERS COMPANY
An Elsevier Science Company

AMIRSYS™

A medical reference publishing company

First Edition

First Printing: November 2002

Composition by Amirsys Inc, Salt Lake City, Utah

Printed by K/P Corporation, Salt Lake City, Utah

ISBN: 0-7216-0034-4

Preface

The **PocketRadiologist™** series is an innovative, quick reference designed to deliver succinct, up-to-date information to practicing professionals "at the point of service." As close as your pocket, each title in the series is written by world-renowned authors. These experts have designated the "top 100" diagnoses or interventional procedures in every major body area, bulleted the most essential facts, and offered high-resolution imaging to illustrate each topic. Selected references are included for further review. Full color anatomic-pathologic computer graphics model many of the actual diseases.

Each **PocketRadiologist™** title follows an identical format. The same information is in the same place - every time - and takes you quickly from key facts to imaging findings, differential diagnosis, pathology, pathophysiology, and relevant clinical information. The interventional modules give you the essentials and "how-tos" of important procedures, including pre- and post-procedure checklists, common problems and complications.

PocketRadiologist™ titles are available in both print and hand-held PDA formats. Currently available modules feature Brain, Head and Neck, Orthopedic (Musculoskeletal) Imaging, Pediatrics, Spine, Chest, Cardiac, Vascular, Abdominal Imaging and Interventional Radiology. 2003 topics will include Obstetrics, Gynecologic Imaging, Breast, and much, much more. Enjoy!

Anne G Osborn MD
Editor-in-Chief, Amirsys Inc

Notice and Disclaimer

PocketRadiologist™
Interventional
Top 100 Procedures

The diagnoses in this book are divided into 8 sections in the following order:

Venous
Dialysis
Arterial
Neuroangiography
Spine & Pain Management
Genitourinary
Chest
Abdomen

Table of Contents

Venous

Dialysis

Arterial

Table of Contents

Neuroangiography

Spine & Pain Management

Genitourinary

Table of Contents

Chest

Abdomen

PocketRadiologist™
Interventional
Top 100 Procedures

VENOUS

Local Anesthetics

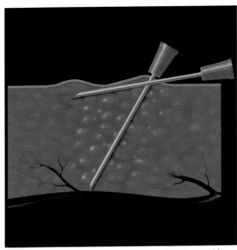

Use of a long needle e.g. 1½ inches, allows same needle to be used for superficial and deeper administration of local anesthetic. Typically a 25, 27 or 30 gauge needle is used.

Key Facts
- Attention to detail in administration of local anesthetic (LA) provides improved pain prevention for patients
- Use 27 to 30-gauge (G) needles
- Inject LA slowly

Pre-Procedure
Indications
- LA is given for almost all interventional radiology (IR) procedures
Contraindications
- Allergy to LA agent
Getting Started
- Things to Check
  - History of allergies to a local anesthetic or other medication
  - Discuss pain prevention with patient
    - Inform patient that you will try to minimize their discomfort
    - Inform patient to notify you when in pain so it may be treated
- Equipment List
  - 1½ inch, 25 to 30 G needle
  - Lidocaine 1% or 2% in plastic container with a rubber stopper
    - Procedure kits often come with lidocaine in a glass ampule because this method of storage provides longer shelf life
    - Downside of glass is need to use filter needle and may cut yourself
  - Local anesthetic should be in a control syringe or at least a different color or size or labeled syringe so that distinct from other syringes
    - Control syringes have finger holes which facilitate one-handed withdrawal of plunger for confirming not intravascular

Local Anesthetics

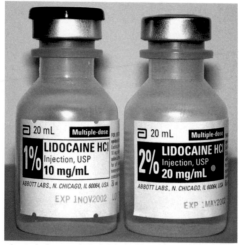

1% lidocaine is used when a relatively large subcutaneous area is infiltrated such as for a chest port. 2% lidocaine is helpful when a relatively small area is infiltrated such as for a biopsy or a pain management spinal injection procedure.

Procedure
Patient Position
- Usually prone or supine with procedure area surrounded by sterile drape

Procedure Steps
- Draw up LA with a short length, 18 G needle
  - Short length, large bore needles allow LA to be drawn up rapidly
  - Inject a few cc of air into plastic container of LA to speed up withdrawal
  - However, do not inject air into glass medication vials as these lack compliance and medication will leak around needle
  - Note number of cc in syringe as will be guide to how much injected
- Connect syringe with 25 to 30 G needle
  - Procedure kits often include short, 25 G needles with light blue hub
  - Preferable to use 1½ inch long, 27 to 30 G needles as these hurt less
  - Added length of 1½ inch needle allows subcutaneous (SQ) and deeper infiltration with same needle
- If plan to also provide intravenous sedation, then give IV medications first
  - Will provide some analgesia before LA needle placed

1% Versus 2% Lidocaine
- In general, if only a small area needs LA use 2% lidocaine
- If need infiltrate more extensive area, such as for chest port placement, 1% lidocaine is preferable to provide more volume

Needle Placement
- Can gently pinch skin with fingers where will insert local anesthetic needle
  - Large, myelinated touch fibers send input to dorsal horn that helps obscure signal from smaller, unmyelinated pain fibers
  - This is consistent with gating theory of pain
- Place LA needle into skin 1 cm away from where will actually puncture or cut for procedure
  - Allows controlled delivery of deep and SQ LA

Local Anesthetics

- o Do not put LA needle straight down at puncture site because as withdraw to make SQ wheal may "backspray" yourself with LA
- Make a good skin wheal as majority of pain receptors located here
- If need to stick needle through skin more than once, go through an area already anesthetized for subsequent needle sticks
- Also inject LA along the planned tract for procedure, including periosteal area when appropriate, because it is innervated
  - o Can use a long, small diameter needle to inject tract
- Important to inject LA very slowly, because rapid injection is painful
- Because LA preferentially blocks small pain fibers, and not larger pressure sensitive fibers, patient will feel pressure during procedure
- "Preemptive analgesia" refers to providing analgesia before procedure starts with goal of preventing pain rather than just treating as it occurs
- Anxiety increases pain and can be decreased by talking in a calm manner
- Intravenous benzodiazepines such as midazolam also decrease anxiety
- Give LA some time to work
  - o A good method is to give LA, and then spend a moment setting up equipment table
  - o Lidocaine skin infiltration usually has taken it's effect within one minute

Additional Options
- Pain of local anesthetic is part due to storage with a weak acid
  - o Can counter by add 1 cc sodium bicarbonate 8.4% per 10 cc lidocaine
- Warming local anesthetic to body temperature can also decrease pain
- Lidocaine wears off in 0.5 to 3 hours, so give additional with long cases

Lidocaine Dosing
- 1% lidocaine contains 10 mg/cc and 2% lidocaine contains 20 mg/cc
- Maximum dose for lidocaine is 4 mg per kg
- Therefore, in a 70 Kg adult (4 mg/kg)(70 kg) = 280 mg is maximum dose
  - o This is 28 cc of 1% lidocaine in a 70 kg adult
- Also remember that LA is absorbed into the vascular system very rapidly in some sites such as intrapleural and intercostal

Lidocaine is Bacteriostatic
- Lidocaine is bacteriostatic and acidic and thus should not be injected into fluid collection, e.g. pleural fluid, that is to be sent for laboratory analysis

Post-Procedure
- Observe patient for signs of LA toxicity

Common Problems & Complications
- Allergic reactions and side effects of LA infiltration for IR are very rare
- Early symptoms of LA toxicity include numbness of tongue, "metallic taste", lightheadedness and dizziness
- These as well as blurred vision and tinnitus can serve as a warning that patient at risk for seizure, respiratory arrest and coma
- Ask patient about symptoms when give relatively large amounts of LA to help identify a potential problem early, and begin treatment with oxygen

Selected References
1. Colaric KB et al: Pain reduction in lidocaine administration through buffering and warming. Am J Emer Med 16:353-6, 1998
2. Fialkov JA et al: Warmed local anesthetic reduces pain of infiltration. Annals of Plastic Surgery 36(1):11-13, 1996
3. Tetzlaff JE: Clinical effects of LA pH adjustments: Review. Anesthesiology Review 20(1):9-15, 1993

Arm Venogram

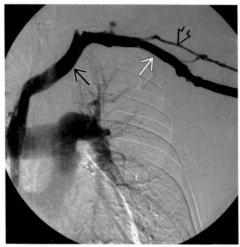

Normal left arm venogram. It shows brachiocephalic vein (black arrow), axillary vein (white arrow) and cephalic vein (open arrow). Note: Normal cephalic vein resembles a hockey stick. Main pulmonary arteries are also opacified.

Key Facts
- Main goal is usually to display venous anatomy of antecubital region and subclavian-brachiocephalic vein junction
- Spot films and tourniquets are used for venogram of arm
- Digital subtraction angiography (DSA) is used for venogram of subclavian and brachiocephalic veins and superior vena cava (SVC)

Pre-Procedure
<u>Indications</u>
- Vein mapping for dialysis graft, cardiac or peripheral vascular surgery
- Nondiagnostic or equivocal ultrasound: For example, to differentiate acute versus chronic deep vein thrombosis (DVT)
- Ultrasound unable to be done due to surgical dressing or painful wound
- Venogram can be requested for more detailed evaluation of subclavian and brachiocephalic veins than provided by ultrasound

<u>Contraindications</u>
- Severe contrast allergy is a relative contraindication
  - Procedure may be done following a steroid and Benadryl prep and with use of nonionic contrast
- Moderate renal failure is a relative contraindication
  - If procedure needs to be done, patient should be hydrated prior to procedure

<u>Getting Started</u>
- Things to Check
  - If antecubital puncture likely to be necessary then check if patient is taking Coumadin
  - If taking Coumadin, check INR
  - Check renal function
  - Performance of this procedure requires at least 2 medical persons, so make sure you have an assistant

Arm Venogram

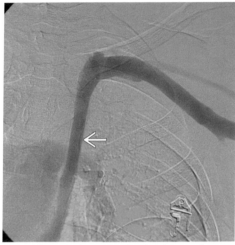

Left arm venogram demonstrates a normal variant left superior vena cava (white arrow). Note: Absence of a left brachiocephalic vein.

- o Clarify indication for study and tailor study to answer relevant clinical question
- o Check if patient has had any previous upper extremity venograms at your institution and try to view these
- Equipment List
  - o 18 or 20-gauge IV Angiocath
  - o Two tourniquets
  - o Angiography procedure table with or without tilting table
  - o Image intensifier of an angiography C-arm is easier to move than that of a multipurpose fluoroscopy room
  - o Quality of fluoroscopy, images and field of view size is more important than having a tilt table
    - Ability to obtain large field of view images is desirable
    - C-arm fluoroscopy with DSA is also desirable
  - o Iodinated contrast 50 to 150 cc

Procedure
Patient Position/Location
- Supine with hand supinated i.e. in anatomical position
Venogram Technique for Arm
- A tourniquet is placed in axilla
  - o And if necessary 2nd tourniquet may be placed just above elbow
- An 18 or 20-gauge IV is started in dorsum of hand if a vein is available
  - o Try to avoid 22 G or smaller IVs
- If patient is a dialysis candidate and has never had a dialysis graft
  - o There is a chance of placing a fistula between radial artery and cephalic vein
  - o Do not put an IV in cephalic vein as this may damage vein
- Usually possible with hand IV to get a good study from forearm to SVC
  - o If venogram from hand vein is not adequate, then may be necessary to place larger IV or make more proximal venous puncture

Arm Venogram

- o Keep in mind that IV may damage vein into which it is placed
- IV is connected to injector tubing which is connected to a 30 to 50 cc syringe filled with contrast
- Contrast is injected and veins of forearm, antecubital region, and upper arm are opacified
  - o Spot radiographs are obtained of these regions
- Several obliquities should be obtained of antecubital region as anatomy can be complex and this is common site for placement of dialysis grafts
- Now arm veins should be full of contrast
- Often axillary vein will be reasonably well opacified at this point and a spot film may be obtained

Venogram Technique for Ipsilateral Chest and SVC
- Blood flow in chest is much more rapid than in arm
- Therefore, DSA is needed to obtain high quality films with injection of contrast from an IV in wrist
- Key is to make use of tourniquet in axilla and contrast which is currently filling arm veins
- Patient is given breathing instructions for upcoming DSA view
- Patient is also told what to expect so will not move when arm is squeezed
- Assistant has job of continuously injecting contrast
- Another person on medical team squeezes forearm and upper arm when DSA screen turns white which signifies that it has completed its initial subtraction and is ready for injection of contrast
- With experience this technique usually provides excellent visualization of subclavian vein, brachiocephalic vein and SVC on first or second attempt
- Usually it is best not to elevate arm as this leads to motion artifact and nondiagnostic DSA
- Rarely, a nonsubtracted venogram with arm elevation will be better

Post-Procedure
Things to Do
- Flush IV with at least 50 cc saline, goal is to rinse contrast out of arm
- Tell patient to flex his/her elbow a few times to further remove contrast
- Confirm with fluoroscopy that IV contrast has been flushed from arm

Common Problems & Complications
- Inadequate opacification of subclavian and brachiocephalic veins
- Extravasation of iodine contrast in hand or forearm
- Contrast allergy

Selected References
1. Shinde TS et al: Three-dimensional Gadolinium-enhanced MR venographic evaluation of patency of central veins in the thorax: Initial experience. Radiology 213:555-60, 1999
2. Menegazzo D et al: Hemodialysis access fistula creation: Preoperative assessment of MR venography and comparison with conventional venography. Radiology 209:723-8, 1998
3. Surratt RS et al: The importance of preoperative evaluation of subclavian vein in dialysis access planning. AJR 156:623-5, 1991

Central Line Complications

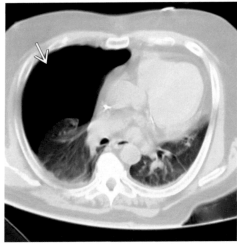

Tension pneumothorax (arrow) after attempted subclavian vein puncture. Initial pneumothorax not visible on supine chest X-ray.

Key Facts
- The most common complications of central venous catheters are infection, bleeding and malfunction due to fibrin sheath or tip malposition

Pre-Procedure
- Check previous catheter history and examine planned area of placement
- Check PT, PTT, INR and platelets
- Check if any previous venous ultrasound or venogram of target area

Procedure
- Arterial puncture and pneumothorax (PTx)
  - Risk is reduced by using ultrasound guidance for venipuncture
- Unable to advance tunneler
  - Immediately after making venipuncture incision, it is helpful to use a mosquito hemostat to "loosen up" tissue where tunneler will need to pass
  - Easier to make tunnel immediately after having accessed the to vein with a 5 French catheter, rather than later when venipuncture incision is more crowded e.g. with a large dilator or peel away sheath
  - Usually when unable to advance thru mid portion of tunnel, it's because tunneler is too superficial or because of scar tissue from previous catheters
  - Can pass a long, narrow hemostat to open up tunnel tract and get thru scar tissue, and also often helps to give more local anesthetic
  - Bend metal tunneler at a right angle to facilitate exit at venipuncture site
- SVC laceration
  - If large dilator passed too forcefully and wire kinks, dilator may pass through wall of SVC
  - Align sheath with wire and twist as advance in small increments
  - Guidewire and dilator should move freely relative to each other

Central Line Complications

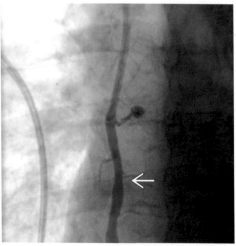

Right subclavian tunneled central venous catheter with tip in right internal mammary vein. Tip location confirmed with injection of iodinated contrast (arrow).

- o Watch dilator advancement under fluoroscopy
- Catheter kink
  - o Use of a venipuncture approach parallel to clavicle with right internal jugular dialysis catheters, decreases likelihood of kink
- Air embolism
  - o Risk reduced by pinching peel away sheath during guidewire removal and catheter introduction
- Kinking of sheath
  - o Can be avoided by only introducing sheath halfway into vein
- Unable to advance catheter thru peel away sheath
  - o Place stiff, angled tip glidewire thru blue lumen to increase pushability of catheter
  - o May need glidewire thru both lumens of catheter
- Malposition of catheter tip
  - o Fluoroscopy facilitates proper tip placement
  - o Catheter tip will characteristically move upward slightly when patient moves from supine to upright
- Post-procedure bleeding
  - o Risk is reduced by not using high dose heparin to initially lock catheter
- Hematoma of port pocket
  - o Obtain hemostasis before inserting port into pocket
  - o More difficult to obtain hemostasis after port sewn into pocket
- Stitch abscess
  - o Tends to occur with silk which is a naturally occurring protein
  - o Silk should not be used for skin
  - o Seldom occurs with monofilament nylon which is a synthetic fiber

Post-Procedure
- If ultrasound used, a postprocedure chest x-ray is usually not obtained
- Can obtain image of catheter position for future reference

Central Line Complications

- If any concern of pneumothorax (PTx), then check with fluoroscopy for large PTx and if none, then obtain chest x-ray to check for small PTx

Common Problems & Complications
- Infection risk is reduced in the following ways
  - Meticulous sterile technique
  - Make skin incisions along Langer's lines
  - Make tunnel entry into venipuncture incision relatively deep so more tissue will cover catheter and easier to suture venipuncture site
  - No showering until catheter site reasonably well healed
- Options for management of catheter infection
  - Obtain blood cultures drawn from peripheral vein and from catheter
  - If suspicion of infection is low and patient has limited venous access, can exchange catheter over a guidewire and send tip for culture
  - When suspicion of catheter infection is moderate to high, can remove catheter and send tip for culture
  - Can sometimes allow a time interval with no indwelling catheter
  - Access needs may require that a new catheter be placed at a different location at same time as infected catheter is removed
  - Central venous catheter infection can lead to sepsis, endocarditis and cervical or lumbar discitis
- Port pocket infection or skin breakdown requires removal of port
- Catheter related internal jugular vein thrombosis is much less common than catheter related subclavian vein thrombosis
- SVC thrombosis precludes placement of dialysis catheter in neck or chest
  - Catheter options include transhepatic, translumbar and femoral
- Partially dislodged catheters can be exchanged over a wire for a new catheter
- If done promptly, new catheters can usually be placed thru the residual tunnel of fully dislodged catheters
- Giant right atrial thrombus
- Arrhythmia rarely occurs with catheter tip in right atrium

Selected References
1. Funaki B: Central venous access: A primer for the diagnostic radiologist. AJR 179: 309-18, 2002
2. Vesely TM: Air embolism during insertion of central venous catheters. JVIR 12:1291-5, 2001
3. Trerotola S et al: Tunneled infusion catheters: Increased incidence of symptomatic venous thrombosis after subclavian versus internal jugular venous access. Radiology 217:89-93, 2000

Chest Ports

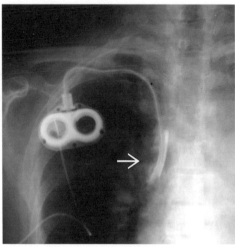

Catheter venography demonstrates a fibrin "sock-sheath" whereby thrombus at catheter tip causes contrast to track retrograde (arrow) along catheter before exiting thrombus/fibrin sheath. Note: This is a double lumen port.

Key Facts
- Right internal jugular vein is usually best site
- Make venipuncture skin nick along Langer's lines
- Make pocket 5-8 mm below skin
- Make tunnel and tunnel exit deep
- Connect port to catheter outside pocket
- Confirm port works before closing pocket
- Use inverted, interrupted, square knots to close pocket

Pre-Procedure

Indications
- Chemotherapy is most common indication
- Long term venous access in patients with difficult access

Contraindications
- Active systemic infection
- Planned radiation to area (relative contraindication)
  - Consider plastic port or place on opposite side
- Multiple prior surgeries which have devascularized area

Getting Started
- Things to Check
  - Bleeding and anticoagulation history
  - Recent chemotherapy or radiation therapy
  - Examine area of planned placement
  - Consider prophylactic antibiotics such as 1 gram of cefazolin IV
  - In patients with penicillin allergy, consider vancomycin
- Equipment List
  - Curved tip and straight tip hemostats
  - Good needle holder and needle pickups
  - Port kit which includes peel away sheath, port and non-coring needle
  - 75 cm long, 0.035" diameter, Amplatz, extra stiff guidewire

Chest Ports

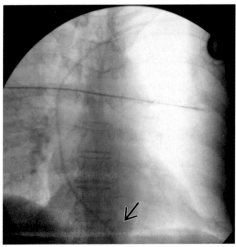

Left subclavian vein chest port catheter (arrow) is too long. Tip could be in RA, RV or coronary sinus.

Procedure

Patient Position/Location
- Supine
- Double prep right chest and neck with alcohol first followed by Betadine

Right Internal Jugular (RIJ) Vein Puncture
- Make sure powder removed from gloves with a wet 4 x 4 gauze
- Make skin nick parallel to Langer's lines as this heals better
- Use a micropuncture needle and ultrasound guidance to puncture RIJ vein
- Advance 0.018" guidewire into SVC and then place 5 French coaxial dilator
- Advance extra stiff wire down into inferior vena cava (IVC)
  - Check monitor for arrhythmia
  - If necessary, use hockey-stick catheter to steer guidewire

Making the Tunnel
- Make port incision about 2 cm caudal to clavicle and parallel to clavicle
- Length of incision determined by size of port
- Easier to make tunnel now, as only a 5 French dilator at vein entry site
- Begin tunnel caudal to clavicle and extend up to skin nick for venipuncture
  - Tunnel extends from port pocket to vein entry site
- Use 1% lidocaine to anesthetize tunnel tract
  - Also creates a plane to facilitate passage of tunneler
- Bend metal tunneler at right angle to facilitate exit from tunnel at neck
- Hemostat can be helpful to open up tunnel tract and get through scar
- Make tunnel and tunnel exit from venipuncture nick deep, as this decreases risk of infection and makes it easier to suture venipuncture nick
- Estimate desired length of catheter tubing by placing it external to patient over location of jugular vein and SVC
- Cut catheter tubing to desired length
- Clamp port end of catheter tubing with hemostat to prevent air embolism when advanced through peel away

Chest Ports

Making Port Pocket
- Open up pocket 5 to 8 mm below skin with a straight tip hemostat
- Try to make only one plane of dissection and gradually expand it
- Make pocket reasonably deep such that there will be enough tissue above it to facilitate suturing the pocket closed
- Check if port fits into pocket
  - Often some additional fibrous strands need to be removed
- Meticulous hemostasis helps to minimize infection risk
- Pocket is packed with gauze while placing peel away sheath

Sheath and Catheter
- Align sheath with wire and twist as advance in small increments
- Guide wire and dilator should move freely relative to each other
- Only insert peel away sheath to halfway point to minimize kinking
- Remove guidewire and sheath dilator
- Pinch sheath with fingers to avoid air embolism as advance catheter
- Optimal tip location is SVC-RA junction

Connecting the Port
- Much easier to connect port to catheter tubing while port is still outside
  - Once port in pocket, it's relatively difficult to connect to tubing
- Can place a "stay" suture in corner of pocket and then thread it thru port base before placing port into pocket
  - Now cut and remove needle from this suture to get needles off procedure field
- Clamp suture with hemostat, but leave suture loose for now so that won't constrict pocket opening
- Confirm port function by aspiration and injection prior to placing port into pocket

Closing Port Pocket and Vein Entry Site
- Close deep layer with inverted, interrupted, square knots using 3-0 Vicryl
- Skin can usually be closed with Steri-Strips
- Subcuticular layer is closed same way, or with running 4-0 Vicryl closure
- If skin sutures required, use 3-0 monofilament, nylon
- Vein entry site can usually be closed with Steri-Strips, if a suture is required, place a single interrupted, inverted, square knot with 3-0 Vicryl

Post-Procedure
- Avoid showers for at least 7 days, sponge baths are okay
- Instruct patient to notify MD if fever, increasing redness of skin over port, opening along suture line, bleeding or other problems related to port
- Give written instructions

Common Problems & Complications
- Infection, sepsis, and subsequent endocarditis or spine infection
- Bleeding or thrombosis of port and adjacent veins e.g. SVC syndrome
- Extravasation of chemotherapy

Selected References
1. Reeves AR et al: Recent trends in central venous catheter placement: A comparison of interventional radiology with other specialties. JVIR 12:1211-4, 2001
2. Kaufman JA et al: Long-term outcomes of radiologically placed arm ports. Radiology 201:725-30,1996
3. Lund GB et al: Outcome of tunneled hemodialysis catheters placed by radiologists. Radiology 198:467-72, 1996

Femoral Vein Puncture

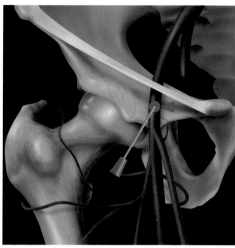

Yellow arrowhead and circle denote target for puncture of common femoral vein. Puncture site is below level of inguinal ligament.

Key Facts
- Right femoral vein is best puncture site for pulmonary angiography, IVC filters, and femoral dialysis catheters
- Common femoral vein is medial to common femoral artery

Pre-Procedure
Indications
- Pulmonary angiography and IVC filters
- Dialysis catheters
- Central line placement during code blue situations
Contraindications
- Infection at planned site
- Thrombosis of entry vein
Getting Started
- Things to Check
  - Previous catheter history
  - Bleeding history, INR, PTT, platelets
  - Examine planned area of placement
    - For signs of previous surgeries or infections
  - Vein with ultrasound prior to prepping target area
- Equipment List
  - Micropuncture kit
  - 0.035" Amplatz, extra stiff, 75 cm long guidewire

Procedure Description
Patient Position
- Supine
Choice of Vein
- Right femoral vein is better entry site for most procedures because right iliac vein straighter and shorter than left

Femoral Vein Puncture

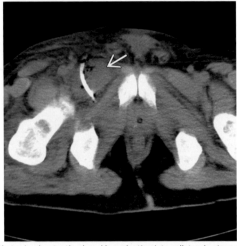

Dialysis catheter inadvertently placed by palpation into collateral vein complicated by **hematoma** *(white arrow) which became infected.*

- Left common iliac vein is also often compressed by adjacent iliac artery
  - Left approach is technically more difficult because tendency of guidewire to go into left ascending lumbar vein
- Fluoroscopy is very helpful for guidewire steering
- Technical ease of right femoral catheter placement relative to left should be remembered for code blue situations where rapid venous access is essential

Ultrasound
- Ultrasound is helpful for femoral punctures
  - Enables visualization of vein, artery and needle
  - Decreases risk of arterial puncture
  - Decreases risk of puncture too high or low
  - Allows choice of favorable approach angle
  - Allows access to vein with fewer sticks
  - Allows visualization if vein is thrombosed

Procedure Steps
- Transducer is placed transverse relative to vein
  - Decrease field of view depth as much as possible to magnify size of vein
  - Bigger target is easier to hit
- Put vein in center of field of view
  - Put needle along center of transducer
  - Maintaining this alignment will facilitate vein entry
- Try to visualize needle from skin entry down to vein
  - Works better than trying to find needle after already advanced inward
  - Needle tip is echogenic
  - Turning down 2D gain will increase visibility of tip
  - Move needle up and down as advance to increase visibility of tip
- Try to puncture center of vein
  - Works better for guidewire advancement

- o If spontaneous blood return not seen, connect 3 cc syringe containing 1 cc saline to needle and check for return
  - o It's easier to work with 3 cc syringe than a 10 cc syringe for this
- Blood return is observed and wire is advanced into vessel
- Advance guidewire into IVC
  - o Avoid wire passage into small, collateral veins
  - o Buckling of wire tip with formation of redundant loop at tip and advancement of guide wire to right atrium both confirm position in IVC
  - o Can use hockey-stick catheter to steer guidewire

Landmark Technique
- Check level with fluoroscopy
  - o Goal is to enter vein at level of middle to lower third of femoral head
- Palpate common femoral artery pulse and "roll" fingers medially to find site for puncture of femoral vein
- Puncture common femoral vein below inguinal ligament
  - o Site of maximal arterial pulse implies correct level to puncture adjacent common femoral vein
- Do not use inguinal crease alone as a landmark as it is sometimes unreliable, especially in overweight persons
- Palpation of anterior-superior iliac spine and pubic symphysis which define inguinal ligament is important in code blue situations where there is no pulse to help identify puncture site
- When wire persistently goes into a collateral vein, a useful maneuver is to just gently advance a 5 French hockey-tip-type catheter thru iliac veins and into IVC
  - o Shape of catheter and its bulkiness help it to stay in main channel of iliac veins and not go into side branches such as ascending lumbar vein

Post-Procedure
Things to Do
- Obtain hemostasis with manual compression

Common Problems & Complications
Complications
- Inadvertent placement of IVC filter into collateral vein parallel to IVC
- Arteriovenous fistula due to arterial puncture
- Hematoma in leg or pelvis

Selected References
1. Zaleski GX et al: Experience with tunneled femoral hemodialysis catheters. AJR 172:493-6, 1999
2. Hertzberg BS et al: Sonographic assessment of lower limb vein diameters; implications for the diagnosis and characterization of deep venous thrombosis. AJR 168: 1253-1257, 1997
3. Abu-Yousef MM et al: Normal lower limb venous doppler phasicity: Is it cardiac or respiratory? AJR 169:1721-5, 1997

Foreign Body Retrieval

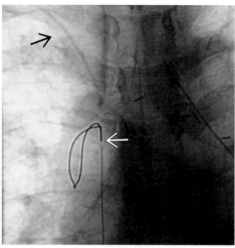

Broken piece of catheter (black arrow) is in right brachiocephalic vein. Loop snare has been placed from the groin and is being positioned. (White arrow) indicates the position of the guiding sheath which has been pulled back to allow expansion of the loop.

Key Facts
- Removal or repositioning of catheters or other foreign bodies
- Foreign bodies within vascular system
  - Catheters, guidewires, pacemaker leads, missile fragments, embolization coils, vascular stents, IVC filters
- Approach depends on location and position
  - Usually femoral venous approach
- Complications
  - Cardiac arrhythmias
  - Cardiac valve damage
  - Papillary muscle damage
  - Vascular perforation
- Most foreign bodies can be removed

Pre-Procedure
Indications
- Foreign body in vascular system
Contraindications
- Unable to perform fluoroscopy
- Severe uncorrectable coagulopathy
Getting Started
- Things to Check
  - Arterial or venous foreign body
  - Plan approach and possible equipment
- Equipment List
  - Sheath to work through
    - Make sure retrieval device will fit through easily
    - Retrieved foreign body should also fit
    - 7-10 French usually appropriate
  - Snare

Foreign Body Retrieval

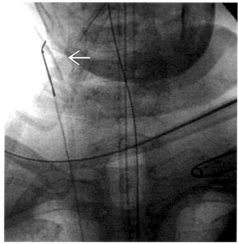

Right subclavian catheter with its tip displaced into right jugular vein. Snare has been placed around catheter tip and closed over catheter tip (arrow) by advancing the guiding catheter. While maintaining traction on the snare and guiding catheter, the tip will be pulled down into the SVC.

- Nitinol gooseneck snare most popular
- Various diameter 5-35mm
- Larger diameters for retrieval in SVC and right atrium
- 90 degree bend relative to shaft of wire
  - Other retrieval devices - stone baskets, grasping forceps, myocardial biopsy forceps, pigtail catheters, deflecting wires
  - Catheters - usually directional - Kumpe, headhunters, Cobra, spinal

Procedure
Patient Position/Location
- Supine
- Good fluoroscopy
- Continuous EKG monitoring, defibrillator

Procedure Steps
- Access into appropriate vascular system
  - Usually right common femoral vein for venous removal
- Place sheath
- Place wire and snare guiding catheter in vicinity of foreign body
- Place snare through the guiding catheter
- Snare advanced until it opens into loop outside of catheter
- Loop passed over the free end of the foreign body
- Wire snare held in position and catheter advanced over wire to tighten the snare around the foreign body
- Holding tension on the snare, the catheter, snare, and foreign body are removed through the vascular sheath

Alternative Procedures/Therapies
- Surgical
  - Rarely needed

Foreign Body Retrieval

- o Occasionally if foreign body is too large to remove percutaneously, a surgical cut-down may be needed as adjunct procedure
- Other
  - o Foreign bodies should be removed whenever possible
  - o Potential complications of foreign bodies
  - o Dysrhythmias, clot formation, embolization, sepsis, vascular or heart perforation with hemorrhage or cardiac tamponade

Post-Procedure
Things to Do
- Standard compression of puncture site

Common Problems & Complications
Problems
- No free end of foreign body available
  - o Pigtail catheter placed over the middle of foreign body and stiffened with tip-deflecting wire
  - o Pulling on pigtail may dislodge ends and allow snaring
- Foreign body too large to pull through sheath
  - o Pull foreign body into proximal sheath and then remove as a unit
  - o Cutdown on venous structure to remove

Complications
- Cardiac arrhythmias
  - o Remove carefully - avoid cardiac valve/papillary muscle damage
- Vascular tear or perforation
  - o Pacemaker wires may be embedded in the myocardium, forceful pulling may result in myocardial tear and pericardial hemorrhage and cardiac tamponade may result

Selected References
1. Gabelmann A et al: Percutaneous retrieval of lost or misplaced intravascular objects. AJR 176:1509-13, 2001
2. Egglin TK et al: Retrieval of intravascular foreign bodies: experience in 32 cases. AJR 164:1259-64, 1995
3. Cekirge S et al: Percutaneous retrieval of foreign bodies: experience with the Nitinol Goose Neck snare. JVIR 4:805-10, 1993

IV Placement

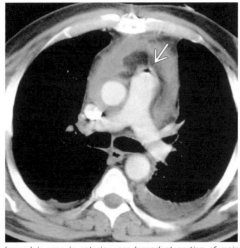

Air bubble (arrow) is seen in anterior, nondependent portion of main pulmonary artery.

Key Facts
- Dorsum of left hand is usually best site for IV's in patients undergoing interventional radiology procedures
- For contrast infusion during IVP's (intravenous pyelograms) or CT's (computed tomography) it is best to put IV in antecubital vein
- Have all ancillary supplies ready before vein is punctured

Pre-Procedure
Indications
- To provide IV access for conscious sedation and other medications
Contraindications
- Unable to palpate or see a vein (relative contraindication)
  - o Ultrasound can be helpful to find a vein
Getting Started
- Things to Check
  - o Coumadin and heparin increase risk of hematoma with antecubital stick
  - o History of renal insufficiency
  - o History of AV shunts or patent ductus
- Equipment List
  - o Tourniquet, 18 to 22-gauge IV, silk tape, alcohol pad or Betadine stick
  - o Local anesthetic with 25 to 30-gauge (G) needle
  - o Flush solution and Hep-lock cap or bag of IV fluids

Procedure
Patient Position
- Supine or seated upright
Equipment Preparation
- Have all ancillary supplies prepared before puncture vein
  - o Tear pieces of tape

IV Placement

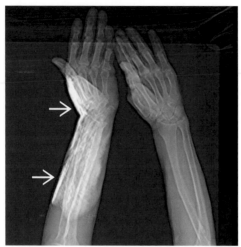

Iodinated contrast extravasation (arrows) occurred during infusion for CT scan. CT topogram image obtained to demonstrate extent of contrast extravasation.

- o Have flush solution or IV fluid tubing within reach
- o Purge IV tubing of air

Choosing Site for IV
- Antecubital region is best site for contrast infusion during CT or IVP
  - o Thick soft tissues have protective effect in event of extravasation
  - o 18 or 20 G is used for rapid infusions such as with CT angiography
  - o 22 G is adequate for routine contrast infusion
- Forearm and wrist are usually best sites for routine inpatient purposes
  - o If will require blood transfusion, preferable to have 18 G or larger IVs
    - With tourniquet placed proximal to increase backflow, these large IV's can also often be used for blood draws
  - o IV's are traumatic to veins and can lead to stenosis or occlusion
  - o Avoid wrist in patients with renal insufficiency as cephalic vein may be used to form fistula with radial artery for dialysis
- For venograms or PICC lines, place IV on side of planned procedure
- For other procedures, usually preferable to have IV placed opposite side
- Dorsum of left hand is usually best site for IVs in patients undergoing interventional radiology procedures
  - o Hand is preferable because more accessible than more proximal areas when patient covered by sterile drape during procedure
  - o Left side is preferable because physician performing procedure is usually on right side of patient when patient is supine
  - o When unsure of where to place IV, check with attending physician
  - o Most inpatients do not like hand IVs as interfere with eating and washing
- Try to avoid placing IVs across joints such as the wrist or phalanges as motion tends to lead to dislodgement or kinking and occlusion

Procedure Steps
- Place tourniquet above antecubital region
- Visually inspect planned site for IV and try to palpate a vein
  - o More important to be able to palpate target vein than to see it

IV Placement

- Prep site with alcohol pad or Betadine stick
- Can inject 1/3 cc of lidocaine 2% to decrease patient discomfort
- Gently move plastic cannula of IV about 1 mm relative to IV needle to make sure plastic part slides smoothly
- Line up long axis of IV with long axis of vein

Needle Placement
- Puncture vein with a short jabbing motion
- When blood return identified, advance needle in an additional 1 or 2 mm
  - So that entire metal needle tip and tip of plastic cannula is within vein
  - This is key step
    - Failure to do this is most common reason for unable to thread cannula
    - If not done, plastic cannula will not go into vein because will collide with anterior wall of vein
- Thread plastic cannula into vein, to hub if possible
- To prevent bleeding, remove tourniquet and press over vein with fingers and then cap with Hep-lock cap or connect to IV tubing
  - Elevation of arm is also useful to prevent bleeding
- Secure IV to skin with silk tape

Code Blue Pearl
- Arm elevation is a fast way to speed central delivery of a medication thru peripheral IV as observed with arm venograms
  - Flushing IV with normal saline is also helpful

Post-Procedure
Things to Do
- Confirm that can inject or infuse IV without extravasation

Common Problems & Complications
- Unable to start IV
- Thrombosis of vein
- Do not readvance needle thru plastic catheter after has been partially moved over needle tip as may shear off plastic
- Extravasation of contrast is usually a minor problem but can be severe:
  - Stop infusion and remove IV
  - Massage contrast out of puncture site, elevate area and apply ice pack
  - Perform neurovascular physical examination of area
  - Obtain spot film or CT scout image to delineate area of extravasation
  - Outline area with soft, marker pen
  - Notify referral service and consult plastic surgery for large volume extravasation or when exam changes are present
- Air embolism can be avoided by purging tubing of air and by completely closing roller clamp during cart to table transfers
  - Otherwise, air from top of IV bag may go into tubing
- In patients that arrive with air in IV tubing, can clear line by placing 16 or 18 G needle into port closest to patient and clamping tubing distal to port

Selected References
1. Lang EV: Treatment to minimize skin or subcutaneous injury if extravasation occurs. AJR 167:277-8, 1996
2. Young RA: Injury due to extravasation of nonionic contrast material. AJR 162:1499, 1994
3. Sistrom CL et al: Extravasation of iopadimol and iohexol during contrast-enhanced CT: Report of 28 cases. Radiology 180:707-10, 1991

Inferior Venacavagram

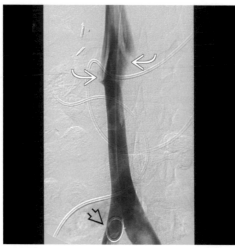

Inferior venacavagram from right internal jugular approach. Note: Bilateral renal veins well seen (curved arrows) and the pigtail catheter (open arrow). The patient had bilateral leg DVT.

Key Facts
- Synonyms: Venogram of inferior vena cava, inferior vena cavography
- Most common indication is with procedure of IVC filter placement
- When imaging for filter placement, check location of Inferior Vena Cava (IVC) bifurcation, and renal veins and for IVC thrombus
- When evaluating a dialysis catheter, check tip location, orientation relative to IVC wall, for presence of fibrin sheath and IVC thrombus

Pre-Procedure
Indications
- Most commonly obtained during IVC filter (IVCF) placement
- Evaluation of femoral dialysis catheter malfunction
- As part of leg venography for DVT
- DVT thrombolysis

Contraindications
- Uncorrectable bleeding diathesis

Getting Started
- Things to Check
  - Bleeding history, platelets, PT, PTT, INR
  - History of any venograms or venous ultrasounds
  - In patients with DVT, try to determine location of DVT
    - Check if right or left common femoral vein is involved
    - Do not puncture thrombosed vein
- Equipment List
  - Entry needle and guidewire
  - 5 French, 65 cm long pigtail catheter with femoral vein puncture and 100 cm length for internal jugular vein (IJV) puncture

Inferior Venacavagram

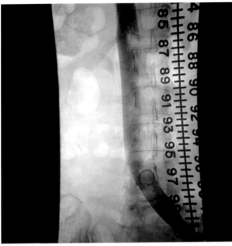

Cavagram from left femoral approach. There was a DVT in the right Common Femoral Vein (CFV). Note: Radiopaque ruler facilitates positioning of IVC filter.

Procedure

Patient Position
- Supine

Femoral Dialysis Catheter Venogram
- Remove heparin from both ports of catheter
- Flush very gently
  - Do not flush forcefully or may dislodge fibrin sheath at catheter tip
- Inject catheter slowly and image with digital subtraction angiography
  - Inject both ports
- Inject with more contrast and more forcefully to evaluate IVC
  - Check for fibrin sheath, catheter tip location, orientation of catheter tip relative to adjacent IVC wall and for IVC thrombus

IVC Venogram Prior to IVCF
- Use ultrasound to check femoral veins before choosing puncture site
- If right common femoral and iliac veins are patent, then it is easiest to place filter from right femoral vein approach
- In general, left femoral vein is less desirable because left iliac veins are relatively angulated and sometimes compressed by right iliac artery
  - Some filters will not be flexible enough to negotiate left side
- However, if right femoral vein is obstructed by thrombus, then left femoral vein is a reasonable choice
  - Right internal jugular vein is other option in this setting
- With use of ultrasound, needle can be visualized as passes into vein
- Landmark technique for puncture of common femoral vein also works well
  - Palpate pulse and roll fingers medially to locate common femoral vein
  - Common femoral vein is medial to common femoral artery
- Use single wall needle and do not put a syringe on it as passed downward
- If artery traversed, will have pulsatile backflow and needle can be withdrawn
- If double wall needle used and/or a syringe placed on hub of a single wall needle, then femoral artery may be traversed unknowingly

Inferior Venacavagram

- o Could lead to a hematoma
- With ultrasound needle can be watched as goes into vein
- Vein is entered and guidewire is passed into vein
- Be gentle as thrombus may be in right iliac vein
  - o Do a hand injection to check that iliac vein appears free of thrombus
- Place a 5 French sheath
- Set table position as desired and lock it into place
  - o Do not move table again for entire procedure
- Worthwhile to advance guidewire all way up to right atrium for absolute confirmation that guidewire is in IVC and not ascending lumbar vein
- Now place pigtail catheter in distal IVC, just proximal to IVC bifurcation

IVC Venogram
- Clamp metal hemostats to sterile drapes over patient at approximate level of upper and lower lumbar spine
  - o These are easier to use as visual landmarks during filter placement than variations in vertebral bodies as guide to for filter placement
- Do a venogram thru coaxial pigtail catheter at iliac vein confluence
- Injection of iodine contrast at 15 cc per sec for a total of 30 cc provides a good cavagram
- Purpose is to define IVC anatomy, check for normal variants, location of renal veins, thrombus in iliac vein or IVC, and IVC diameter

Anatomical Variants
- Left IVC
- Duplicated IVC
- Large diameter IVC, e.g. more than 28 mm
- Retroaortic left renal vein
- Circumaortic left renal vein
- Extrinsic compression of IVC by mass lesions

Alternatives to Iodinated Contrast
- CO_2
- Gadolinium
- Selective catheterization of renal veins and contralateral iliac vein can serve as landmarks to guide IVC filter placement
  - o Can obtain a spot film of catheter at each location and can place a radiopaque hemostat to correspond to level

Post-Procedure
Things to Do
- Bed rest x 6 hours following IVC gram and placement of IVC filter
- If IVC gram done thru indwelling femoral dialysis catheter, then post-procedure bedrest is not required

Common Problems & Complications
- Puncture site complications such as hematoma
- Injury to common femoral artery

Selected References
1. Urban BA et al: Three-dimensional volume-rendered CT angiography of the renal arteries and veins: Normal anatomy, variants, and clinical applications. Radiographics 21:373-86, 2001
2. Dewald CL et al: Vena cavography with CO_2 versus with iodinated contrast material for inferior vena cava filter placement: A prospective evaluation. Radiology 216:752-7, 2000
3. Bass JE et al: Spectrum of congenital anomalies of the inferior vena cava: Cross-sectional imaging findings. Radiographics 20:639-52, 2000

IVC Filter Placement

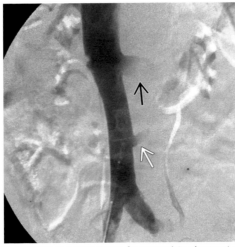

Inferior vena cavagram is a requirement for appropriate placement of IVC filter. (Black arrow) indicates left renal vein. (White arrow) indicates circumaortic left renal vein.

Key Facts
- Procedure definition: Placement of IVC filter to protect against pulmonary emboli
- Clinical setting triggering procedure: Deep venous thrombosis or pulmonary emboli, patient cannot be anticoagulated
- Best procedure approach: Right common femoral vein, right jugular vein
- Most feared complication(s): Migration of filter to right heart, incorrect deployment, access site or IVC thrombosis, IVC perforation
- Expected outcome: Placement of IVC filter in appropriate location

Pre-Procedure
<u>Indications</u>
- Deep venous thrombosis and/or pulmonary emboli
  - Contraindication to anticoagulation
  - Complication of anticoagulation
  - Failure of anticoagulation
  - Prophylactic placement-controversial

<u>Relative Contraindications</u>
- Severe uncorrectable coagulopathy

<u>Getting Started</u>
- Things to Check
  - Ultrasound documenting thrombosis
  - Previous CT of abdomen – evidence of cava anomalies
- Equipment List
  - One-wall needle or micropuncture set if using jugular approach
  - 5 Fr dilator, standard angiographic wire
  - IVC filter
    - Greenfield, Bird's Nest, Vena-Tech, Nitinol, Tulip, Trapease
    - Delivery system appropriate for the venous approach
    - Jugular, femoral or brachial vein

IVC Filter Placement

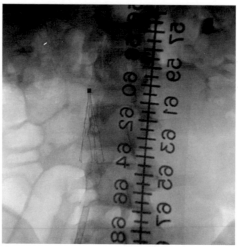

Placement of Greenfield filter in infrarenal IVC. Note: Marking ruler placed under patient to aid in correct placement.

- o Ultrasound if doing jugular or brachial vein approach
- o 5 Fr pigtail or Omni flush catheter preferably with size markers

Procedure
<u>Patient Position/Location</u>
- Supine, good fluoroscopy

<u>Equipment Preparation</u>
- Make sure you know workings of the filter device, read directions!
- Type of filter less important than correct usage
- Make sure have filter type for planned approach
- Once sure of approach and placement, prep filter as necessary

<u>Procedure Steps</u>
- Choose access- usually right femoral vein or right jugular vein
- Filters also placed from left femoral, left jugular, some via brachial vein
- If jugular approach use ultrasound to access vein
- Femoral approach after puncture, place 5 Fr dilator and inject contrast, verify no clot in iliofemoral system
- Place pigtail catheter in low IVC at venous confluence
- IVC gram
  - o Demonstrate patency of IVC, presence of clots
  - o Assess size
  - o Position and number of renal veins
  - o Renal veins or IVC anomalies – duplicated IVC, circumaortic renal veins
- To evaluate anomalies selective catheterization may be required
- Measure size of cava, make sure not too large for planned filter
- Place wire, may be specific wire with filter
- Dilate venotomy if necessary
- Position filter in correct position
- Placement optimally infrarenal IVC, tip of filter just below renal veins
- Deploy filter, image to make sure it has deployed properly
- Remove filter carrier and compress venotomy site

IVC Filter Placement

Alternative Procedures/Therapies
- Surgical
  - Filters can be placed surgically via cutdown in femoral or jugular vein
  - Caval ligation or plication can be performed, very uncommon

Post-Procedure
Things to Do
- If possible, anticoagulated, will minimize chance of filter thrombosis

Common Problems & Complications
Problems
- Cava too large for filter
  - Use Bird's Nest, okay up to 45 mm
  - Place a filter in both iliac veins
- Duplicated IVC
  - Place filter in both IVC channels
- Circumaortic left renal vein
  - Place filter caudal to lower segment of vein, avoids potential conduit for clots
- Clot in IVC
  - Place filter in suprarenal IVC from a jugular or brachial approach
- History of severe contrast reaction
  - CO2 or gadolinium for IVC gram

Complications
- Severe
  - Migration of filter – cava too large for filter, migration to right atrium or pulmonary arteries
  - Misplacement into inappropriate vessels
  - IVC thrombosis potentially life-threatening; phlegmasia cerulea dolens; thrombosis above filter leading to pulmonary emboli
  - IVC perforation usually well tolerated, perforation of bowel can cause severe morbidity
  - Tilting of filter or incorrect opening –may require second filter
- Other complications
  - Access site thrombosis
  - Dislodgement or entrapment of filter by catheters or guidewires
  - Filter fracture

Selected References
1. Savin MA et al: Placement of vena cava filters: factors affecting technical success and immediate complications. AJR 179:597-602, 2002
2. Athanasoulis CA et al: Inferior vena cava filters: review of a 26-year single center clinical experience. Radiology 216:54-66, 2000
3. Kaufman JA et al: Operator errors during percutaneous placement of vena cava filters. AJR 165:1281-7, 1995

Jugular Vein Puncture

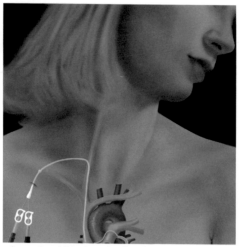

Right jugular is punctured 1 to 4 cm distal to clavicle. Catheter tunnel exit site is infraclavicular.

Key Facts
- Right internal jugular vein (RIJv) is best puncture site for transjugular liver biopsy (TJLBx), transjugular intrahepatic portal-systemic shunt (TIPS) and for dialysis catheters
- Low, anterior, perpendicular approach is used for dialysis catheters
- High, anterior, parallel approach is used for TJLBx and TIPS
- Pneumothorax, bleeding and carotid puncture are main complications
- Use ultrasound and micropuncture needle with 0.018" guidewire
- Exchange for extra stiff guidewire then placed into IVC
- Align sheath with wire as advance in small increments

Pre-Procedure
Indications
- TJLBx, TIPPS and IVC filters
- Dialysis catheters, tunneled Groshong catheters and portacaths
Contraindications
- Infection at planned site
- Occlusion of entry vein (relative contraindication)
Things to Check
- Previous catheter history
  - Bleeding history, INR, PTT, platelets
  - Examine planned area of placement
    - Check for signs of previous catheters, surgeries or infections
  - If multiple previous catheters, then check vein with ultrasound prior to prepping target area
- Equipment List
  - Micropuncture kit
  - 0.035" Amplatz, extra stiff, 75 cm long guidewire

Jugular Vein Puncture

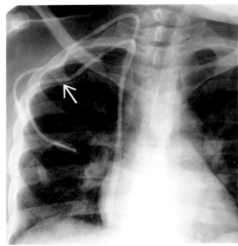

2 Piece permanent dialysis catheter placed with 2 punctures in RIJV. With a single piece catheter, lower puncture site is preferable. Tunnel extends out to an infraclavicular exit site (white arrow).

Procedure

<u>Patient Position/Location</u>
- Supine
- Procedure table should be parallel to ground
- Trendelenburg positioning is not necessary, but maybe helpful

<u>Ultrasound</u>
- Ultrasound should be used for jugular punctures
  - Enables visualization of vein, artery and needle
  - Decreases risk of pneumothorax
  - Decreases risk of carotid puncture

<u>Procedure Steps</u>
- Puncture perpendicular to vein for catheters
- For catheter placement make skin nick parallel to Langer's lines
  - Improves healing and cosmesis
  - Use a low, anterior approach perpendicular to RIJV
- Point needle bevel towards SVC
  - Helps steer guidewire towards SVC
- Transducer is placed transverse relative to vein
  - Increases length of needle visible
  - Decrease field of view depth as much as possible to magnify size of vein
  - Bigger target is easier to hit
- Put vein in center of field of view
  - Put needle along center of transducer
    - Facilitates needle visualization and vein entry
- Try to visualize needle from skin entry down to vein
  - Works better than trying to find needle after already advanced inward
  - Needle tip is echogenic
  - Turning down 2D gain will increase visibility of tip
- Try to puncture center of vein

Jugular Vein Puncture

- o Works better for guidewire advancement
- If spontaneous blood return not seen, connect 3 cc syringe containing 1 cc saline to needle and check for return
- Blood return is observed and guidewire is advanced into vessel
- Advance 0.018" guidewire into SVC
- Place 5 French coaxial micropuncture dilator
- Exchange for 75 cm long, Amplatz extra stiff wire
- Advance extra stiff wire down into IVC
  - o Check ECG monitor for arrhythmia
  - o Can use 5 French, 40 cm hockey stick catheter to steer guidewire
  - o LAO projection moves atrium off spine to show wire

Placing Large Sheaths
- Most dangerous part of procedure
  - o If dilator passed too forcefully and wire kinks, dilator may pass through wall of SVC
- There are several keys to completing this part of procedure safely
  - o Use an Amplatz, extra stiff guidewire
  - o Place guidewire down into IVC
  - o Line up long axis of dilator sheath with guide wire
  - o Advance in small increments, watch under fluoroscopy
  - o Use a gentle, rotatory, side-to-side motion as sheath advanced over guidewire
  - o Gently pull wire back and forth slightly as sheath advanced
    - This is an essential step
    - Guidewire and dilator should move freely relative to each other
    - As long as sheath moving freely relative to wire, then wire is not kinked and all is well
- Main site of resistance is when sheath step-off relative to sheath dilator contacts fascial tissue around vein
- Once sheath component is in vein, resistance will decrease

Post-Procedure
- Observe for at least one hour
- If any concern of pneumothorax, then view lung apex with fluoroscopy
  - o Place chest tube if large, symptomatic pneumothorax present
- If clinical symptoms suggest pneumothorax yet none seen on fluoroscopy of lung apex, then obtain upright AP expiration and inspiration CXR
  - o Keep patient in department until have viewed CXR

Common Problems & Complications
- Pneumothorax
- SVC laceration
- Arrhythmia
- Jugular vein thrombosis

Selected References
1. Trerotola SO et al: Tunneled infusion catheters: increased incidence of symptomatic venous thrombosis after subclavian versus internal jugular venous access. RJ 217:89-93, 2000
2. Sasadeusz KJ et al: Tunneled jugular small-bore central catheters as an alternative to peripherally inserted central catheters for intermediate-term venous access in patients with hemodialysis and chronic renal insufficiency. RJ 213:303-6, 1999
3. Trerotola SO et al: Outcome of tunneled hemodialysis catheters placed via the right internal jugular vein by interventional radiologists. RJ 203:489-95, 1997

Leg Venogram

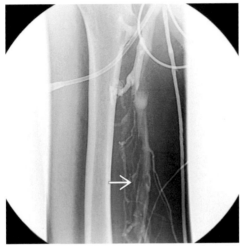

DVT of right superficial femoral vein due to right common femoral vein dialysis catheter. Note: Thrombus seen as filling defect along venous valve cusp (arrow).

Key Facts
- Most common indication is to check for deep vein thrombosis (DVT)

Pre-Procedure
<u>Indications</u>
- Nondiagnostic or equivocal ultrasound
  - For example, to differentiate acute versus chronic DVT
- Ultrasound unable to be done due to surgical dressing
- Vein mapping for dialysis graft, cardiac or peripheral vascular surgery
- Evaluation of iliac veins

<u>Contraindications</u>
- Severe contrast allergy is a relative contraindication
- Moderate renal failure is a relative contraindication
  - If must be done, patient should be hydrated

<u>Getting Started</u>
- Things to Check
  - Angiography procedure table with or without tilting table
  - Quality of fluoroscopy, spot films and field of view size are more important than having a tilt table
  - Iodinated contrast 100 to 200 cc
- Equipment List
  - Two tourniquets
  - 21 and 23-gauge butterfly needles are usually best
    - At times a 22-gauge Angiocath is helpful
  - Angiography procedure table with or without tilting table

Procedure
<u>Patient Position</u>
- Supine with table flat, i.e. parallel to floor
- Obtain scout AP radiographs of lower leg, thigh, and pelvis

Leg Venogram

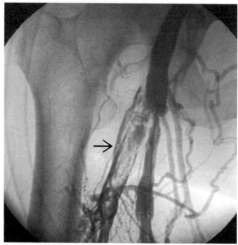

DVT (arrow) is seen as filling defect in deep femoral vein. Note: "Tram track" appearance of contrast outlining the thrombus.

Equipment Preparation
- If using a tilt table, put non-studied foot on a block of wood so that it will be weight bearing
- Prefer standard angiography non-tilt tables over tilt tables because they are faster and easier
  - Faster because fluoroscopy tends to be better and can view images in real time
  - Easier on patient, because patients do not have to support all their weight on one foot

Procedure Steps
- Place a tourniquet above knee and ankle
- Start a butterfly needle or Angiocath in foot
  - Tape it securely
  - Leave some slack in butterfly tubing
  - It's helpful to loop tubing through web space of toes
- Applying mild pressure or "tapping" while wiping with an alcohol pad over dorsum of foot can improve visualization of veins
- Dependent positioning of foot may increase distention of foot veins
- Ultrasound is helpful when foot veins are difficult to palpate
  - Use high frequency linear transducer
- Manually compressing foot edema for a minute or two and then letting up pressure and quickly searching for a vein is sometimes helpful
- Inject test dose of saline to make sure it does not extravasate
- Inject contrast and obtain images of calf, thigh, pelvis and IVC

Calf Views
- In upper calf-knee area there are a lot of overlapping veins
  - Therefore get views in at least two different obliquities
- Obtain delayed or magnified images of questionable areas

Thigh Views
- A single AP view is adequate for mid to upper thigh veins

Leg Venogram

Pelvis and IVC
- A single AP view is adequate for pelvis-lower IVC region
- Fill calf and thigh veins with contrast
- Optimize position of image intensifier over pelvis and lower IVC
- Compress common femoral vein to impede flow of contrast
- Simultaneously elevate leg manually
  - o Squeeze calf
  - o And have an assistant release tourniquets
  - o Continue injecting contrast throughout entire process
  - o Now take film(s) while this is occurring
- Goal is to obtain film during maximal opacification
- In some patients, simply compressing the calf will provide adequate opacification of iliac veins with DSA

Post-Procedure
Things to Do
- Flush IV with at least 50 cc saline
- Goal is to rinse iodinated contrast out of leg veins
- Tell patient to move his/her feet up and down like stepping on gas pedal to further remove iodine contrast
  - o Confirm with fluoroscopy that contrast gone from leg veins

Common Problems & Complications
Problems
- Extravasation of contrast in foot
Complications
- Contrast allergy
- Irritation of leg veins by iodinated contrast which was more of a problem in past when nonionic contrast was used

Selected References
1. Johns CM et al: US-guided venipuncture for venography in the edematous leg. Radiology 180:573, 1991
2. Bhargava R et al: Contrast venography in patients with very edematous feet: Use of transdermal illumination to aid in vein puncture. Radiology 179:583, 1991
3. LeVeen RF et al: Pressure-infusion venography of leg with remote-control fluoroscopy. Radiology 138:730-1, 1981

PICC Line Ultrasound

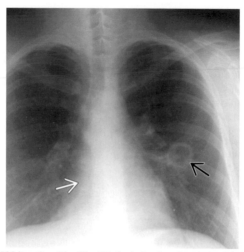

Left arm PICC line placed for IV antibiotics to treat cavitary lesion (black arrow) of lung abscess. Tip of PICC (white arrow).

Key Facts
- PICC line is most common long-term venous catheter
- Main reason is provides similar benefits as centrally placed catheter, but with decreased risk
- PICC line can remain in place for months

Pre-Procedure
Indications
- Long term IV access

Contraindications
- No accessible veins in arms

Getting Started
- Things to Check
  - Please see "PICC Line Venogram" diagnosis
- Equipment List
  - Micropuncture kit with 21-gauge needle and 0.018" guidewire
  - PICC line kit which usually includes PICC line, stiffener guidewire for PICC line and peel away sheath
  - 3-0 monofilament nylon (e.g. Ethilon) suture

Procedure
Patient Position
- Supine with arm extended at elbow
- Arm is prepped circumferentially from upper bicep level to 10 cm distal to antecubital crease
- Tourniquet is placed high in axilla
  - Tourniquet must be tight
  - Makes vein more taut and thus easy to puncture

Choice of Vein
- Usually best vein to enter is basilic, several cm above antecubital crease
  - Because it is usually relatively large and far from arteries

PICC Line Ultrasound

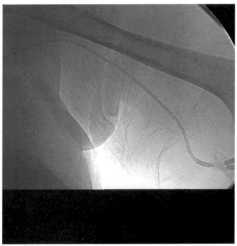

Left arm PICC line. Position catheter exit for patient comfort and so that nurse will have easy access.

- Second choice vein is brachial
- In general, try to avoid putting PICC lines into cephalic vein
  - Because it tends to go into spasm
  - Cephalic vein also tends to thrombose

Ultrasound Guidance
- Scan veins and choose a target site for entry
  - Veins will be readily compressible
  - Artery will be pulsatile and resistant to compression
- Administer just enough local anesthetic (LA) to prevent pain with needle placement
  - Too much LA can obscure ultrasound visualization of vein
  - Can give more LA after guidewire is in vein
- Make a nick in skin with a #11 scalpel
  - Easier to make nick now than after guidewire placement
  - If make nick after guidewire, make sure in continuity with guidewire, otherwise, won't be able to place dilator
- Gently spread skin nick with mosquito hemostat
- Magnify vessel as much as possible by decreasing field of view depth
  - Bigger target is easier to hit
- Transducer footprint should be perpendicular-transverse to target vein
- Put target vein into center of scanning field of view
  - That way if needle is center of transducer at skin level, then it is more likely will continue down into vein
- Goal is to enter target vein while avoiding brachial artery
- Turn down 2D gain
  - Will make needle tip more visible, since tip is echogenic
- If needle is difficult to visualize
  - Try to follow it from when it first enters skin
  - Move it back and forth
  - Turn down 2D gain even further
- Make a slight jabbing motion as poke needle into vein

- o This facilitates a one wall puncture
- Follow with guidewire and then peel away sheath
  - o Make sure skin nick is wide enough for sheath
  - o This is most common reason for difficulty in advancing sheath
- If encounter some resistance while placing dilator and peel away sheath
  - o Make sure skin nick in continuity with guidewire
  - o Make sure guidewire is not kinked
  - o Align sheath with wire and twist as advance in small increments
  - o Guidewire and dilator should move freely relative to each other
  - o If tip of dilator is bent or damaged then get another dilator

Tip Placement
- Distal tip is cut to appropriate length with conventional open tip catheters
- Hub end is cut to appropriate length with Groshong catheters
- Place tip of catheter at superior vena cava-right atrial junction
- This relates to when a patient elevates his/her arm,
  - o While supine, catheter may move inward several cm
  - o If catheter goes into right ventricle, it may cause an arrhythmia
- Confirm ability to aspirate blood
- Fill (also referred to as locking catheter) catheter with flush solution
  - o Most catheters are locked with heparinized saline or saline
  - o Check guidelines for catheter type being placed
- Suture catheter to skin with 3-0 monofilament nylon
- Cover with sterile dressing

Post-Procedure

Things to Do
- Observe patient for evidence of complications
- Monitor blood pressure, pulse and arm for hematoma

Common Problems and Complications

- Inadvertent dislodgement
- Hematoma and infection
- Thrombosis of catheter or arm veins
- Injury to brachial artery
- Injury to median nerve can occur with brachial vein PICC
- Arrhythmia is rare

Selected References
1. Hoffer EK et al: Prospective randomized comparison of valved versus nonvalved peripherally inserted central vein catheters. AJR 173:1393-8, 1999
2. Polak JF et al: Peripherally inserted central venous catheters: Factors affecting patient satisfaction. AJR 170:1609-11, 1998
3. Sofocleous CT et al: Sonographically guided placement of peripherally inserted central venous catheters: review of 355 procedures. AJR 170:1613-6, 1998

PICC Line Venogram

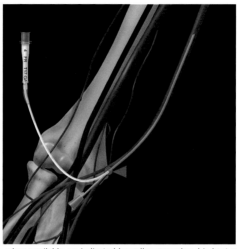

Basilic vein, when available, as indicated by yellow arrowhead is best vein for PICC line placement followed by brachial veins.

Key Facts
- PICC lines are most common long-term venous catheter
- Main reason for popularity is similar benefits as a centrally placed catheter, but with decreased risk

Pre-Procedure
<u>Indications</u>
- Intravenous antibiotics for osteomyelitis or endocarditis
- Hyperalimentation
- Chemotherapy

<u>Contraindications</u>
- No accessible veins in arms
- Occlusion of bilateral subclavian veins (relative contraindication)
- Renal failure on hemodialysis (relative contraindication)

<u>Getting Started</u>
- Things to Check
  - Ask if patient is right handed or left handed
    - Most patients will prefer PICC placed in nondominant arm
  - If a recent infection in arm, then go to opposite side
  - If has indwelling IV, this is helpful for venography
  - Check if any previous PICC lines or venograms
  - If known subclavian occlusion, then go to opposite side
  - If INR is above 1.5, or platelets less than 40,000, then try to correct if possible
    - If procedure needs to be done with abnormal INR, then use a superficial forearm vein as these are easy to compress
    - Use arm elevation and a slightly compressive, noncircumferential dressing for hemostasis
  - Check creatinine if intend to use venography
- Equipment List
  - Micropuncture kit with 21-gauge needle and 0.018" guidewire

PICC Line Venogram

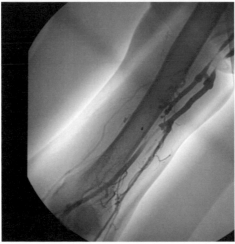

Right arm venogram is done with contrast injection from an IV in the hand and with a tourniquet placed in axilla. First choice for PICC placement is usually basilic vein followed by brachial vein.

o PICC line kit which usually includes PICC line, stiffener guidewire for PICC line and peel-away sheath
o Groshong-type tip is a valve which blocks passive reflux into catheter
  ▪ Allows Groshong catheter to be flushed with saline rather than heparinized saline
o Open-tip catheters are typically flushed with heparin flush
o 3-0 monofilament nylon (e.g. Ethilon) suture

Procedure
Patient Position
- Supine with arm extended at elbow
- Arm is prepped circumferentially from upper biceps level to 10 cm distal to antecubital crease
- Tourniquet is placed high in axilla
Equipment Preparation
- Flush PICC line
Choice of Vein
- Basilic is best vein because usually large and far from arteries or nerves
- Second choice is a brachial vein
  o However, it is near median nerve and rarely a PICC line placed here can be associated with irritation of median nerve, especially if a hematoma occurs
- Cephalic vein is last choice because superficial and tends to spasm
Venogram Technique
- Tourniquet must be tight
  o If loose, vein will collapse and guidewire will not advance into vein
- Venogram of arm is obtained by injection of contrast thru IV in hand
- Choose target site for venipuncture
- Administer local anesthetic and make a nick in skin with #11 scalpel
- Gently spread skin nick with a mosquito hemostat

PICC Line Venogram

- Put target vein into center of fluoroscopy field of view
- Technique is like "spear fishing"
  - Put target vein into center of fluoroscopy field of view
- Magnify as much as possible and collimate
- Needle is advanced towards vein which visibly indents upon contact
  - Gently poke into vein
  - Try not to go thru posterior wall or contrast will extravasate
- Advance 0.018" guidewire into vein and then place peel away sheath
- Place tip at SVC-RA junction
- Suture catheter to skin with 3-0 monofilament nylon
- Flush catheter with flush solution

PICC Line Exchange
- PICC lines with damaged, irreparable hubs and malfunctioning PICC lines can be exchanged
- Key to procedure is to use an angled-tip, 0.018" glidewire for the exchange
- Make sure external portion of indwelling catheter is very well prepped
  - Can be dipped, soaked in Betadine
- Use scissors to cut off external part of indwelling PICC
  - Discard it
- Place 0.018" glidewire thru indwelling PICC
- With Groshong PICC's, a little force is needed to overcome valve at tip
- Remove indwelling PICC completely
- Place new sheath over 0.018" glidewire
- Place new PICC

PICC Line Removal
- Simply remove PICC and hold pressure for 10 minutes
  - Can be done on wards or even as an outpatient
  - Does not need to be done in radiology department

Post-Procedure
Things to Do
- Check patient for evidence of complication, such as hematoma

Common Problems & Complications
- Bleeding can usually be managed with manual compression
- Inadvertent dislodgement
- Infection
- Thrombosis of arm or central veins
- Injury to brachial artery
- Injury to median nerve

Selected References
1. Hoffer EK et al: Prospective randomized comparison of valved versus nonvalved peripherally inserted central vein catheters. AJR 173:1393-8, 1999
2. Polak JF et al: Peripherally inserted central venous catheters: factors affecting patient satisfaction. AJR 170:1609-11, 1998
3. Chait PC et al: Peripherally inserted central catheters in children. Radiology 197:775-8, 1995

Subclavian Vein Puncture

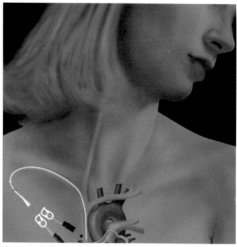

Illustration shows typical course of a right subclavian vein catheter. Note: Blue port of catheter is located laterally as this helps place catheter tip sidehole away from wall of SVC or RA.

Key Facts
- Right internal jugular vein (RIJv) is best puncture site for dialysis catheters and chest port catheters
- Subclavian vein is punctured when RIJv is occluded or not available for other reasons such as infection, neck surgery or tracheostomy
- There are 3 basic techniques for subclavian vein puncture: 1) Ultrasound, 2) Venography, 3) Landmark palpation
- Ultrasound guidance with a micropuncture needle and 0.018" guidewire is most common method
- Exchange for extra stiff guidewire which is then placed into IVC
- Align sheath with wire as advance in small increments
- Pneumothorax, bleeding and arterial puncture are main complications

Pre-Procedure
Indications
- Dialysis catheters, tunneled Groshong catheters and portacaths
  - Especially when the RIJv is not available and/or fluoroscopy and ultrasound are not available as these facilitate jugular puncture

Contraindications
- Infection at planned site
- Occlusion of entry vein

Getting Started
- Things to Check
  - Previous catheter history
  - Bleeding history, INR, PTT, platelets
  - Examine planned area of placement
    - Check for signs of previous catheters, surgeries or infections
  - If had previous catheters, then check vein with ultrasound prior to prepping target area
- Equipment List

Subclavian Vein Puncture

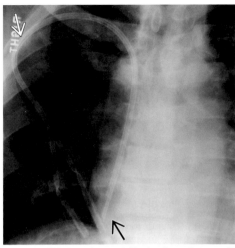

Right subclavian vein dialysis catheter. Unlike jugular catheters, with subclavian catheter will not feel catheter on top of clavicle. Jugular vein was occluded in this patient. White arrow denotes tunnel exit site of catheter. Black arrow points to tip of catheter in right atrium.

- o Micropuncture kit with 21-gauge needle and 0.018" guidewire
- o 0.035" Amplatz, extra stiff, 75 cm long guidewire

Procedure

Patient Position
- Supine
- Procedure table should be parallel to ground
  - o Trendelenburg positioning is not necessary

Ultrasound Benefits
- Ultrasound is helpful for subclavian vein puncture
  - o Enables visualization of vein, artery and needle
  - o Decreases risk of pneumothorax
  - o Decreases risk of arterial puncture

Ultrasound-Guided Procedure Steps
- Transducer may be placed transverse or longitudinal relative to vein
  - o Decrease field of view depth as much as possible to magnify vein
    - Bigger target is easier to hit
- Put vein in center of field of view and needle along center of transducer
  - o Facilitates needle visualization and vein entry
  - o Try to puncture center of vein
  - o Works better for guidewire advancement
- Try to visualize needle from skin entry down to vein
  - o Works better than trying to find needle after already advanced inward
  - o Needle tip is echogenic
    - Turning down 2D gain will increase visibility of tip
- Make skin nick parallel to Langer's lines
  - o Improves healing and cosmesis
- Needle bevel should face upwards
  - o Facilitates guidewire advancement into subclavian vein

Subclavian Vein Puncture

- If spontaneous blood return not seen, connect 3 cc syringe containing 1 cc saline to needle and check for return
- Blood return is observed and guidewire is advanced into vessel
  - Advance 0.018" guidewire into SVC
- Place 5 French coaxial micropuncture dilator
- Exchange for 75 cm long, Amplatz extra stiff wire
  - Advance extra stiff wire down into IVC
  - Check ECG monitor for arrhythmia
  - Can use 5 French, 40 cm hockey-stick catheter to steer guidewire
  - LAO projection moves atrium off spine to show wire

Venogram Guided Procedure Steps
- Iodinated contrast is injected thru ipsilateral arm IV
- Hemostat placed over 1st or 2nd rib to line up puncture route where axillary vein or subclavian vein pass over these ribs
  - Concept is that needle will hit rib, not lung, if passes thru vein
- Superimpose needle tip and hub and advance into vein

Landmark Palpation Procedure Steps
- Palpate suprasternal notch and infraclavicular space
- Advance needle just inferior to junction of middle and lateral third of clavicle aimed in direction of suprasternal notch

Post-Procedure

Things to Do
- Observe for at least one hour
- If any concern of pneumothorax, then view lung apex with fluoroscopy
  - Place chest tube if large, symptomatic pneumothorax present
- If clinical symptoms suggest pneumothorax yet none seen on fluoroscopy of lung apex, then obtain upright AP expiration and inspiration CXR
  - Keep patient in department until have viewed CXR

Common Problems & Complications

- Difficulty advancing dilators may occur with steep approach angle
- Pneumothorax is rare with ultrasound guidance
  - However, in large patients, even with ultrasound, the subclavian vein can be difficult to see
- Arterial puncture may lead to hematoma or arteriovenous fistula
- Arrhythmia
- SVC laceration
- Subclavian vein stenosis or occlusion
  - Much more common than catheter related jugular vein thrombosis
- Pinch-off syndrome with catheter fracture

Selected References
1. Trerotola SO et al: Tunneled infusion catheters: Increased incidence of symptomatic venous thrombosis after subclavian versus internal jugular venous access. RJ 217:89-93, 2000
2. Muhm M et al: Supraclavicular approach to subclavian/innominate vein for large-bore central venous catheters. Am J of Kidney Dis 30:802-8, 1997
3. Trerotola SO et al: Outcome of hemodialysis catheters placed via the right internal jugular vein by interventional radiologists. RJ 203:489-95, 1997

Transjugular Liver Biopsy

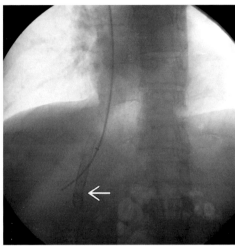

Transjugular liver biopsy done as part of preoperative evaluation for liver transplantation. Note: The patient has a TIPS stent (white arrow).

Key Facts
- Transjugular liver biopsy involves obtaining access to right jugular vein, catheterizing right hepatic vein (RHV) and directing a slotted needle anteriorly into hepatic parenchyma to obtain a core biopsy specimen

Pre-Procedure
Indications
- Liver biopsy in patients contraindicated or high risk for percutaneous biopsy due to coagulopathy or thrombocytopenia or due to massive ascites
- Preoperative evaluation of liver transplant candidates
- Diffuse liver disease

Contraindications
- Unable to obtain consent

Getting Started
- Things to Check
  - Bleeding history, platelets, PT, PTT, INR and hemoglobin
  - Check prior imaging studies such as ultrasound, CT and MRI
  - Check right hepatic vein patency and orientation relative to IVC and liver
  - Check for any tumors or cysts in right lobe of liver anterior to RHV
  - Check overall liver size and whether displaced upward
  - Check posterior extent of RHV relative to vertebral body
    - This is useful reference for when check catheter position in RHV on lateral view of fluoroscopy
- Equipment List
  - Multipurpose Glidecath
  - Amplatz, extra-stiff guidewire 145 cm long, 0.035" diameter
  - Iodinated contrast
  - Cook Company Quick Core Coaxial Transjugular Liver Biopsy Kit
    - 7 French sheath

Transjugular Liver Biopsy

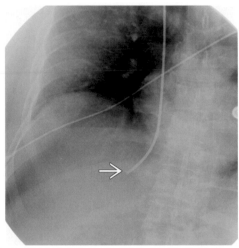

Transjugular liver biopsy done in a patient with diffuse liver disease, no focal lesion on CT and abnormal clotting parameters. White arrow points to biopsy needle.

- 19-gauge slotted needle with a trigger mechanism for firing and a 20 mm throw length which is helpful for obtaining nice core specimens

Procedure
Patient Position
- Supine
  - EKG tracing, oxygen saturation and pulse should be monitored throughout procedure
Procedure Steps
- Use ultrasound guidance to puncture right internal jugular vein
- Puncture parallel to long axis of right internal jugular vein
- Place 9 French sheath
Right Hepatic Vein Catheterization
- Use a multipurpose Glidecath
- Right hepatic vein tends to enter IVC very high, almost at level of diaphragmatic hiatus
- Probe with catheter along right lateral and posterolateral IVC wall to enter RHV
- Once catheter tip is in RHV, it usually can be gently advanced further into vein without a guidewire
- Check catheter location on AP and lateral fluoroscopy
- If it is in RHV, it will be quite posterior
  - This is desirable
- If it is in middle hepatic vein, it will be relatively anterior
- A hepatic vein venogram is obtained at this time
  - Helps confirm that catheter is in right hepatic vein
  - Can also document appearance of middle hepatic vein on AP view
- Right and middle hepatic veins can have very similar appearances on AP view

Transjugular Liver Biopsy

Needle Placement
- Place 0.035", 145 cm long Amplatz extra stiff guidewire into RHV
- Exchange catheter for biopsy kit sheath
  - Some physicians preassemble the device and already will have 7 French sheath in place around Glidecath and will simply exchange over guidewire for biopsy needle
- Maintain constant downward pressure on sheath while it is in RHV
  - Otherwise, will tend to move back out into IVC due to cardiac and respiratory motion
  - This can lead to cardiac arrhythmia or tamponade
- Advance needle gently, under direct fluoroscopic observation down into RHV
- Direct needle anteriorly and obtain a specimen
  - Slotted inner stylet is advanced into liver parenchyma
  - Outer cutting cannula is then activated with trigger button mechanism
- Usually 2-3 specimens are obtained

Specimen Preparation
- Discuss with pathology department at your hospital
- Specimens are placed into formalin
- If viral studies are needed, these can be placed in saline

Post-Procedure
Things to Do
- Observe patient for 6 hours

Common Problems & Complications
- Unable to obtain stable catheter position in hepatic vein
- Failure to obtain diagnostic specimen
- Cardiac arrhythmia e.g. due to prolapse of catheter or sheath into right ventricle
- Cardiac tamponade e.g. due to prolapse of needle into right atrium
- Bile duct or gallbladder injury by needle
- Hepatic artery injury by needle e.g. with formation of pseudoaneurysm or arteriovenous or arterioportal fistula
  - May present with hemobilia and melena
- Liver capsule puncture and hemoperitoneum

Selected References
1. Roche CJ et al: Intrahepatic pseudoaneurysm complicating transjugular biopsy of the liver. AJR 177:819-821, 2001
2. Banares R et al: Randomized controlled trial of aspiration needle versus automated biopsy device for transjugular liver biopsy. JVIR 12: 583-7, 2001
3. Middlebrook M et al: Improved method for transjugular liver biopsy. JVIR 10:807-9, 1999

Radiation Protection

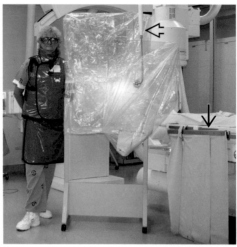

Lead shield (black arrow) on procedure table protects legs. Ceiling shield (open black arrow) protects upper body. Door shield protects both. Technologist has lead glasses, thyroid shield, lead vest and lead skirt/wraparound (moves weight bearing away from back).

Key Facts
- Try to minimize radiation exposure to patient and yourself
- Always inquire about pregnancy in female patients of reproductive age

Pre-Procedure
Indications
- All procedures which involve fluoroscopy

Contraindications
- None

Getting Started
- Things to check
  - Check that radiation protection devices are available for procedure
    - E.g. remember to bring leaded eyeglasses to procedure area

Equipment List
- Leaded eyeglasses
  - Can significantly decrease radiation exposure to eyes
  - Downside is that some are heavy and uncomfortable
  - Shop around to find a pair that is comfortable enough that you will actually wear them
  - Chronic radiation exposure can cause cataracts
- Thyroid shield
  - Decreases risk of radiation-induced thyroid cancer
- Lead apron
  - It is best to buy your own lead apron
  - Take good care of it
  - If folded repeatedly and mishandled, will develop cracks thru which you will be exposed to radiation
  - Can check apron for cracks by placing on an angiography table and viewing with fluoroscopy

Radiation Protection

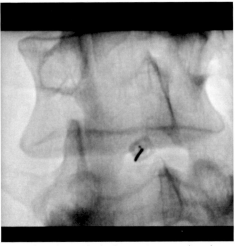

Tight collimation as shown here with a lumbar puncture procedure, decreases radiation exposure to patient and physician.

- o Two-piece aprons have a wraparound "kilt-like" component that puts weight on hips instead of back
    - This is important if do a lot of procedures and/or have a "bad back"
- Connector tubing for contrast injection
    - o Connector tubing is helpful because it increases distance between you and x-ray beam during hand injections of contrast
- Power injector
    - o In general, for obtaining angiography images, it is preferable to use a power injector rather than perform hand injections
    - o Power injection usually produces better blood vessel opacification
    - o However, hand injections have advantage of being much faster to perform
- Lead drapes attached to angiography table
    - o Hang down from angiography table
    - o Decrease radiation exposure to personnel's legs and gonads
- Lead drape attached to fluoroscope
    - o Typically are found on fixed fluoroscopy units used for barium studies
    - o When working in these rooms, use these when possible
- Lead sliding door
    - o This is a leaded glass door on wheels
    - o It is used during angiography procedures while doing hand injections of contrast
    - o Also, if a nurse or anesthesiologist needs to be in room during procedure, they can often sit behind one of these
- Lead shield from ceiling
    - o These are leaded glass shields which hang from ceiling on a metal articulated arm
    - o Although at times cumbersome, can significantly decrease radiation exposure to physician during interventional procedures

Radiation Protection

Procedure

Patient Position
- Depends on type of procedure

Procedure Steps
- SID
  - SID stands for source to image distance
  - Keeping image intensifier (II) close to patient decreases scatter
- Collimation
  - Metal collimators decrease area exposed to x-ray beam
  - Collimate whenever possible
  - Significantly decreases x-ray exposure to patient and physician
- Distance
  - Radiation exposure is determined by inverse square rule
    - If 2 feet away from beam instead of 1 foot away, your exposure will be 4 times less (1/1 versus 1/2x2=1/4)
  - Bottom line is, further are from beam, less the exposure
- Pulsed fluoro
  - Utilizes intermittent pulses of radiation
  - Can lead to lower exposure to patient and physician
- Keep your hands out
  - Try to keep hands out of path of x-ray beam
  - Putting hands in beam greatly increases radiation dose to hands
    - This can lead to skin cancer
- Try to minimize duration of fluoroscopy during procedures
  - Prolonged duration of fluoroscopy is most common cause of excessive radiation exposure to patient

Long Procedures
- During procedures such as TIPS and embolization, prolonged fluoroscopy may be necessary
- Try to collimate and angle beam to avoid excess radiation to a single area

Post-Procedure

Things to Do
- Depends on type of procedure

Common Problems & Complications
- Cataracts
- Skin erythema and painful ulceration
- Hair loss
- Skin cancer

Selected References
1. Wagner LK et al: Management of patient skin dose in fluoroscopically guided interventional procedures. JVIR 11:25-33, 2000
    Ito H et al: Analysis of radiation scatter during angiographic procedures: Evaluation of a phantom model and a modified protection radiation system. JVIR 10:1343-50, 1999
    hope TB: Radiation-induced skin injuries from fluoroscopy. Radiographics 16:1195-9,1996

PocketRadiologist™
Interventional
Top 100 Procedures

DIALYSIS

Dialysis Catheter Exchange

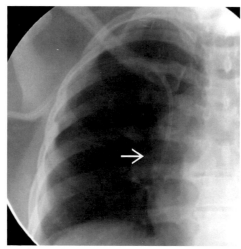

Initial dialysis catheter with tip at SVC-RA junction is no longer functional with flows of around 150 cc per minute and frequent intermittent occlusions. Note: The tip of catheter (arrow).

Key Facts
- Dialysis catheter exchange refers to changing an indwelling hemodialysis catheter (I-HDC) for a new catheter over a guidewire
- Most common indication is malfunction of I-HDC due to fibrin sheath
- New catheter usually placed with different tip orientation or overall length
- Examine catheter with fluoroscopy to assess cause of malfunction
- Palpate cuff before administering local anesthetic (LA)
- Remove heparin from indwelling catheter
- Use 0.035" angled tip, stiff glidewire
- Use meticulous sterile technique

Pre-Procedure
Indications
- Malfunction of I-HDC due to malposition or fibrin sheath
Contraindications
- Grossly infected catheter e.g. with purulence
Getting Started
- Things to Check
  - Check that attempts have been made to salvage I-HDC
    - Arm elevation
    - Turning head to side
    - Seated, supine and decubitus positioning
    - Digital pressure on catheter
    - Reversing I-HDC ports for withdrawal and return of blood: Causes increased recirculation, but may provide adequate dialysis
    - TPA filling and possibly infusion of catheter
  - Bleeding history and PT, PTT, INR if on heparin or Coumadin
  - History of previous dialysis catheters
  - Previous venograms or venous ultrasounds of upper extremity
  - Discuss procedure plan with referral service e.g. nephrology

Dialysis Catheter Exchange

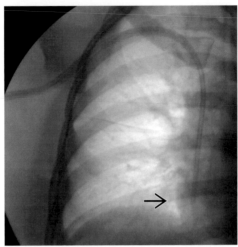

Indwelling catheter was removed over 0.035 stiff glidewire passed thru catheter and down into distal IVC. A new catheter was then placed deeper into the right atrium (arrow) and flows were better than 300 cc per minute by hand-syringe test.

- o Check when patient last dialyzed and when next appointment
    - ▪ Typical schedules are Mon-Wed-Fri or Tue-Thu-Sat
    - ▪ If dialysis excessively delayed, patient may become fluid overloaded and hyperkalemic
- Equipment List
    - o HDC with a cuff
        - ▪ Typically same length or slightly longer than I-HDC
    - o 0.035" angled tip, stiff glidewire
        - ▪ Stiff glidewires provide more support than regular glidewires
        - ▪ Angled tip helps for steering glidewire into inferior vena cava

Procedure
<u>Patient Position</u>
- Supine
- Perform a meticulous prep
    - o I-HDC can be soaked in Betadine
<u>Procedure Steps</u>
- Visually inspect I- HDC for infection
- Check length
    - o If 36 cm in length, might want to put in a longer catheter e.g. 40 cm
    - o If 36 cm long and already in mid right atrium then don't put in longer catheter which will likely go in too far
- Look at catheter under fluoroscopy
    - o Check if kinked
    - o Check tip position e.g. proximal superior vena cava (SVC) (not good), mid SVC (suboptimal), distal SVC (acceptable), SVC/RA junction (good), upper RA (good), mid RA (usually good if supine)
- Check tip orientation and how behaves during cardiac cycle
    - o If cleft side (contains red port endhole) contacts SVC or RA wall, implies more likely to form fibrin sheath and not function well

Dialysis Catheter Exchange

- Consider reversing orientation of red and blue hubs of new catheter outside patient relative to orientation of I-HDC red and blue hubs
  - o May lead to better tip endhole orientation
- Palpate cuff
  - o This way if catheter not easy to remove from tunnel exit site, will know where to cut down on cuff
  - o If give LA before palpate cuff, may be difficult to locate cuff
  - o Usually, if I-HDC has been in place less than 3 weeks, it is very easy to remove and often can be pulled without need for any dissection
- Remove heparin from I-HDC
  - o Dialysis catheters are often primed/locked with heparin at a concentration of 5,000 units per cc
  - o Each lumen typically holds about 1.5 cc or 7,500 units of heparin
  - o Gently tugging on catheter as withdraw syringe plunger facilitates aspiration of heparin
  - o Failure to remove heparin may lead to prolonged bleeding

Catheter Exchange

- Pull or dissect I-HDC so that cuff is just outside skin entry site of tunnel
- Place 0.035" angled-tip glidewire thru blue port and advance into IVC
  - o Placing stiff glidewire well into IVC facilitates advancing new HDC
  - o May need 2nd glidewire thru red port to increase pushability
- Remove I-HDC over glidewire
- Place new HDC, with tip orientated to optimize flow, over guidewire
- Advance to desired location e.g. tip in lower SVC or upper RA

Test That New HDC has "Good Flow"

- Desirable flow rate is greater than or equal to 300 cc/minute
- Use a 10 cc syringe to check flow rate
  - o Do not use any other size syringe
  - o Connect syringe to catheter and briskly pull back plunger
  - o If can pull 10 cc in 2 seconds, correlates with 300 cc/minute
  - o Thus, goal is to be able to pull back 10 cc within 2 seconds
- Lock catheter with heparinized saline e.g. at a concentration of 100 to 1000 units heparin per cc
  - o Do not use 5,000 units/cc because associated with increased risk of bleeding

Post-Procedure

Things to Do

- Observe patient 1 hour or send to dialysis unit

Common Problems & Complications

- Infection
- Dislodgement
- Bleeding
- Recurrent fibrin sheath

Selected References

1. Garofalo RS et al: Exchange of poorly functioning tunneled permanent hemodialysis catheters. AJR 173(1):155-8, 1999
2. Drusak R et al: Replacement of dialysis catheters thru preexisting tunnels. JVIR 9(2):321-7, 1998
3. Robinson D et al: Treatment of Infected tunneled dialysis catheters with guidewire exchange. Kidney Int 53(6): 1792-4, 1998

Dialysis Catheter Removal

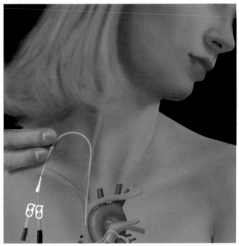

Dialysis catheter cuff is palpated prior to administration of local anesthetic. Therefore cuff location is known in event that need to cut down directly to cuff.

Key Facts
- In case a cutdown to cuff is necessary, palpate cuff prior to giving local anesthetic
  - Otherwise cuff will become nonpalpable
- Use meticulous sterile technique to avoid false positive bacterial cultures

Pre-Procedure
Indications
- Infected catheter
- Sepsis of unknown origin with catheter as possible source
- Catheter malfunction refractory to salvage
- Catheter no longer needed

Contraindications
- Unable to obtain dialysis access elsewhere
  - Make sure other access option is available before removing catheter

Getting Started
- Things to Check
  - How long ago catheter was placed
    - If less than 2 weeks ago, then most likely cuff is not yet adherent and catheter will slide right out
    - This means removal can be done without a significant amount of dissection and that procedure will proceed quickly
- Equipment List
  - Curved tip hemostat, number 11 scalpel and sterile scissors
  - Lidocaine 1% or 2% local anesthetic
    - If available, 2% lidocaine is preferable as it provides a longer, more dense duration of analgesia
  - 10 cc syringe and 25 to 32-gauge needle for administration of local anesthetic
  - 10 cc syringe for aspiration of heparin from catheter prior to removal

Dialysis Catheter Removal

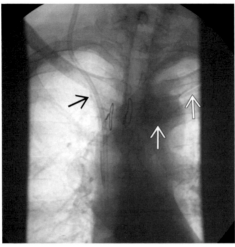

Malfunctioning temporary left subclavian catheter (white arrows) was removed. New right external jugular tunneled catheter (black arrow) was placed. Right internal jugular vein is occluded. Patient is scheduled for left arm dialysis graft placement.

- o Sterile container for placement of potentially infected catheter to send to laboratory
  - ▪ A sterile urine specimen type cup can be used for this purpose

Procedure

Patient Position/ Location
- Supine
- Procedure usually done on angiography table, but can be done at bedside
  - o Don't need to use fluoroscopy, so don't need to wear lead

Prepping Catheter
- A meticulous prep is important to avoid false positive bacteria cultures
- It can be difficult to thoroughly prep external portion of a catheter
  - o This can be dipped in a basin containing liquid Betadine and then covered with a sterile towel
  - o Do not touch this part of catheter except to remove heparin
  - o If inadvertently touched, then change your gloves
- You must palpate catheter cuff before giving local anesthetic
  - o Otherwise cuff will be obscured and may be difficult to find later if a cutdown to cuff is needed
  - o Most often cuff is near tunnel exit site
  - o However, sometimes it is up near vein entry site at end of a long tunnel and if in place for over 2 months may require a cutdown directly above cuff

Heparin Removal
- Dialysis catheters are typically loaded with concentrated heparin flush
- If released into patient, this may cause prolonged post-procedure bleeding
- Remove heparin from both lumens of indwelling catheter

Dialysis Catheter Removal

- o If unable to initially obtain flow, then tug and release catheter and try again to aspirate with a syringe
- o This almost always works
- Now clamp catheter about 1 cm from skin entry site
- Remaining external portion of catheter should be covered with a sterile towel and not touched again

Catheter Removal
- Be generous with local anesthetic
- A lot of scar tissue forms around a catheter and can be quite painful when catheter is pulled
- Next step is to see if catheter can be pulled out easily
- Give a gentle tug
- If in for more than 3 months, there is usually a lot of scar tissue
- Removal requires completely dissecting cuff away from scar tissue
- Dissect cuff free using a hemostat
- Individual fibrous strands can be pulled from cuff by using hemostat
- With more experience at catheter removal, you will find that it is much faster and easier to use a scalpel for sharp dissection to free up cuff
  - o Be careful while doing this to not cut catheter
  - o Inner part of catheter may embolize into patient

Sending Catheter for Microbiology Analysis
- Send inner part, (part that was inside patient), to microbiology lab for gram stain and culture
- Catheter can be cut into 5 cm long segments and placed into a sterile urine specimen type container and then sent to microbiology

Post-Procedure
Things to Do
- Obtain hemostasis
  - o Hold pressure over vein entry site for 10 minutes
  - o Factors which will increase likelihood for bleeding are increased duration in patient, larger diameter catheters, chronic steroid therapy, femoral catheters and high venous pressure such as occurs in subclavian catheters placed downstream to a patent dialysis graft
  - o Sit patient upright to decrease venous pressure in jugular and subclavian veins which is helpful for maintaining early post-procedure hemostasis

Common Problems & Complications
- Catheter breakage which may embolize into patient
- Air embolism
- Bleeding and hematoma formation

Selected References
1. Kohli MD et al: Outcome of polyester cuff retention following traction removal of tunneled central venous catheters. Radiology 219:651-4, 2001
2. Funaki B et al: Radiologic placement of tunneled hemodialysis catheters in occluded neck, chest or small thyrocervical collateral veins in central venous occlusion. Radiology 218: 471-6, 2001
3. Trerotola Scott et al: Tunneled infusion catheters: Increased incidence of symptomatic venous thrombosis after subclavian versus internal jugular venous access. Radiology 217: 89-93, 2000

Dialysis Graft Angioplasty

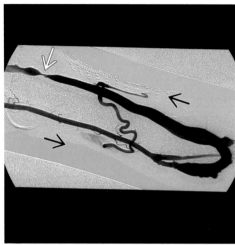

Dialysis fistula (black arrows), indicate the flow of the blood through the fistula. The (white arrow) indicates the stenosis in the venous outflow. Small veins arising from the fistula indicate this is a fistula rather than a graft.

Key Facts
- Treatment of venous stenosis occurring in the venous outflow
- Presentation
  - Elevated venous pressures, abnormal flow velocities during dialysis, decreased thrill, high pitched bruit over the venous outflow
- Direct puncture of the dialysis fistula/graft
  - Venous angiogram
  - Dilatation of venous stenosis with angioplasty balloon
- Complications
  - Thrombosis, rupture of vein
- Angioplasty very successful
  - High rate of recurrence in 3-6 months, repeat angioplasty warranted

Pre-Procedure
Indications
- Dysfunctional fistula/graft
  - High venous pressures, abnormal flow velocities
- Physical examination
  - Decreased thrill, high pitched bruit, difficult hemostasis post dialysis

Contraindications
- Severe contrast reaction, severe coagulopathy, infection

Getting Started
- Things to Check
  - Allergies, coagulation status, evidence of graft infection
  - Previous studies for sizing of balloon
- Equipment List
  - One wall needle, or micropuncture set, Terumo/other hydrophilic wire, 5 French dilator
  - Angioplasty balloon
    - Size chosen after evaluation of venous outflow

Dialysis Graft Angioplasty

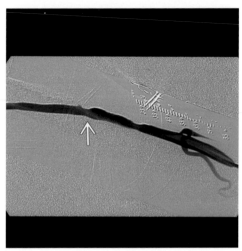

Post angioplasty site (arrow) with a good angiographic result. The stenosis has been relieved. Note: The measuring device (partially subtracted) just above the vein, this device can be helpful in determining the appropriate size for the balloon.

- 5-6 French, short shaft (40 cm), 4 cm long balloon (usually 6-9 mm), high pressure balloon
  o Short sheaths for dialysis
  o Heparin, sedation

Procedure
Patient Position/Location
- Position so whole fistula/graft and outflow to level of major draining vein (usually superior vena cava) can be imaged

Procedure Steps
- Sterile preparation and draping of entire fistula/graft
- Start at site close to arterial anastomosis, give anesthesia
- Needle directed towards venous anastomosis
- Grasp fistula/graft between thumb and forefinger of one hand
- Puncture fistula/graft, place wire and then dilator into the fistula/graft
- Keep dilator tip relatively close to puncture site initially
- Inject contrast, film fistula/graft, venous outflow to level of right atrium
- Compress fistula/graft and inject contrast to opacify arterial anastomosis
- Stenosis in venous outflow
  o Choose appropriate angioplasty balloon
  o Give 2,000-3,000 units of heparin
  o Dilate stenosis with inflation device, maintain high pressure for 2 min
  o Release and repeat inflation
- Reevaluate stenosis
- If still narrowed, and no pain with inflation, repeat with larger balloon
- Treat other stenoses in venous outflow with appropriately sized balloon
- When good angiographic result
  o Patient going to dialysis, exchange catheter for dialysis sheath
  o If patient not going to dialysis, remove catheter, hold **gentle** pressure

Dialysis Graft Angioplasty

Alternative Procedures/Therapies
- Radiologic
  - If stenosis can not be relieved then consider stent placement
    - Make sure large enough balloon placed with high enough pressure to treat stenosis
    - Avoid stent placement that will limit surgical options
    - Stent placement likely to increase recurrent stenoses, monitor closely
- Surgical
  - Surgical revision
    - Direct revision of stenosis
    - Jump graft to region higher up in the vein

Post-Procedure
Things to Do
- Consider antiplatelet medications
  - Aspirin
    - Will not prevent recurrent stenosis
    - May help to avoid thrombosis when stenosis recurs
- Educate patient
  - The stenosis will recur
  - Difficult hemostasis post dialysis sign of significant stenosis
  - Consider scheduled appointment in 3-4 months

Things to Avoid
- No tight dressings around fistula/graft
- Avoid excess pressure on fistula/graft

Common Problems & Complications
Post Angioplasty Residual Stenosis
- Usually not a large enough balloon
  - If no discomfort with inflation, use larger balloon
  - Avoid stent unless pain with inflation, stenosis **clearly** elastic

Complications
- Rupture of vein
  - Usually too large a balloon
  - Position balloon across rupture, inflate for 5 minutes, reimage
  - Place self-expanding stent to divert flow past tear
  - If continued leak, may need to thrombose fistula/graft, refer to surgery for placement of new fistula/graft
- Thrombosis of fistula/graft
  - Less likely with fistula than with graft
  - Treat with thrombolysis (see chapter on dialysis graft thrombolysis)

Selected References
1. Beathard GA: Angioplasty for arteriovenous grafts and fistulae. Semin Nephrol 22: 202-10, 2002
2. Turmel-Rodrigues L et al: Interventional radiology in hemodialysis fistulae and grafts: a multidisciplinary approach. Cardiovasc Intervent Radiol 25: 3-16, 2002
3. Rundback JH et al: Venous rupture complicating hemodialysis access angioplasty: Percutaneous treatment and outcomes in seven patients. AJR 171: 1081-4, 1998

Dialysis Graft Thrombolysis

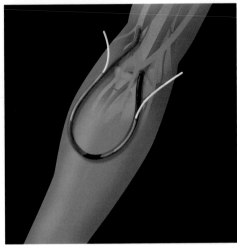

Loop graft that demonstrates cross catheter technique. First catheter placed from the arterial end directed towards venous anastomosis. If able to pass venous stenosis, then second catheter placed from the venous end of graft towards arterial end.

Key Facts
- Treatment of occluded dialysis graft
- Patient presents with occluded dialysis graft
- Catheter placement of thrombolytic agent into graft
- Complications
  - Bleeding from graft
  - Sepsis
  - Pulmonary emboli
  - Arterial embolus
- Thrombolysis usually very successful
  - Reveal underlying venous stenosis, treat with angioplasty

Pre-Procedure

Indications
- Thrombosed dialysis graft

Contraindications
- Contraindication to thrombolysis
- Infection of graft, severe coagulopathy, severe contrast reaction
- Inability to pass a wire across the venous stenosis

Getting Started
- Things to Check
  - Evidence of infection, allergies, coagulation status
  - Previous angiographic studies of graft
- Equipment List
  - One wall needle, or micropuncture set
  - Terumo/other hydrophilic wire helpful to pass tight stenosis
  - 5 French dilators
  - Multi-side-hole catheter for administering thrombolytic
  - Angioplasty balloon

Dialysis Graft Thrombolysis

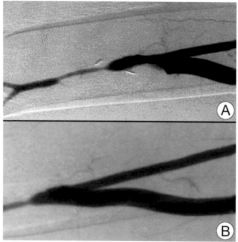

(A) Once thrombolysis performed evaluate venous outflow and angioplasty venous stenosis. (B) Then evaluate arterial end, and if resistant clot, sweep with occlusion/ thrombectomy catheter.

- Occlusion balloon/Fogarty catheter, remove resistant clot at arterial anastomosis
- Short sheaths to allow dialysis post procedure
- Thrombolytic (tPA, reteplase), heparin, conscious sedation

Procedure
Patient Position/Location
- Angiographic or fluoroscopy room
- Position so whole graft, outflow to right atrium can be imaged

Procedure Steps
- Sterile preparation and draping of entire graft
- Start at site close to arterial anastomosis, give anesthesia
- Needle directed towards venous anastomosis
- Grasp graft between thumb and forefinger of one hand
- Puncture graft, there may be no blood return
- Place wire through the needle, should pass easily, follow course of graft
- Place dilator over the wire into the graft
- Inject contrast, demonstrate venous outflow
- Exchange for multi-sided-hole catheter
- Evaluate venous outflow to the level of the right atrium
- Second catheter placed from venous end towards arterial end
- Thrombolysis using thrombolytic – pulse 0.2-0.4 cc q 20 seconds
  - TPA 2 mg in 20 cc of NS divided between the two catheters
  - Reteplase 3-5 units in 20 cc of NS divided between the catheters
  - Heparin 2-3,000 units intravenously
- After administering thrombolytic
  - Identify venous stenosis and treat per dialysis angioplasty chapter
  - Evaluate arterial anastomosis
- Arterial anastomosis commonly has resistant clot

- o Place occlusion balloon/Fogarty balloon catheter just beyond clot into arterial inflow
- o Inflate balloon and pull back across clot
- o Enough pressure in balloon to give some resistance, not enough to disrupt anastomosis
- When good angiographic result
  - o Patient going to dialysis, exchange catheter for dialysis sheath
  - o If patient not going to dialysis, remove catheter, hold **gentle** pressure

Alternative Procedures/Therapies
- Radiologic
  - o Lyse and wait/lyse and go, please see chapter on this topic
  - o Thrombectomy devices
- Surgical
  - o Thrombectomy
  - o Angiographic evaluation and angioplasty following thrombectomy

Post-Procedure
Things to Do
- Immediate dialysis with full anticoagulation
- Consider antiplatelet and anticoagulants
- Consider scheduled appointment in 3-4 months, for angiographic follow-up, possible prophylactic balloon dilatation

Things to Avoid
- No tight dressings

Common Problems & Complications
Unable to Pass Venous Stenosis
- Abandon procedure
  - o Thrombolysis will cause lysis, without outflow, bleeding at puncture sites

Bleeding from Previous Puncture Sites
- Manually compress
- Angioplasty venous stenosis as quickly as possible

Unable to Thrombolyse Graft
- Reassess technique
- Possible infected thrombus-resistant to thrombolysis

Arterial Clot Lodges in Graft or Venous Outflow
- Treat with angioplasty balloon to fragment

Complications
- Arterial anastomotic clot embolizes into artery
  - o Prevention - avoid angioplasty of arterial clot
  - o Place wire past embolus, advance occlusion balloon over wire, drag embolus back into graft
  - o If not in major artery, patient may not need anything
  - o Heparinize patient

Selected References
1. Falk A et al: Thrombolysis of clotted hemodialysis grafts with tissue-type plasminogen activator. JVIR 12: 305-11, 2001
2. Falk A et al: Reteplase in the treatment of thrombosed hemodialysis grafts. JVIR 12: 1257-62, 2001
3. Roberts AC et al: Pulse-spray pharmacomechanical thrombolysis for treatment of thrombosed dialysis access grafts. Am J Surg 16: 221-6, 1993

Dialysis Graft Lyse and Wait

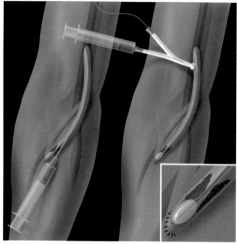

Puncture of arterial end of graft with needle or Angiocath. Manual occlusion of arterial and venous ends of graft and injection of thrombolytic agent.

Key Facts
- Treatment of occluded dialysis graft
- Patient presents with occluded dialysis graft
- Direct puncture of graft, instill thrombolytic agent
- Complications
  - Bleeding from graft
  - Injection of thrombolytic outside graft
  - Sepsis
  - Pulmonary emboli
  - Arterial embolus
- Thrombolysis usually successful
  - Reveal venous stenosis, treat venous stenosis with angioplasty

Pre-Procedure
Indications
- Thrombosed dialysis graft
Contraindications
- Infection of graft, severe coagulopathy, severe contrast reaction
Getting Started
- Things to Check
  - Evidence of infection, allergies, coagulation status
  - Previous studies of graft
- Equipment List
  - Needle, Angiocath, or micropuncture set
  - Terumo/other hydrophilic wire for crossing venous stenosis
  - Angioplasty balloon
  - Occlusion balloon /Fogarty catheter, remove clot at arterial anastomosis
  - Sheaths to allow dialysis post procedure
  - Thrombolytic (tPA, Reteplase), heparin, conscious sedation

Dialysis Graft Lyse and Wait

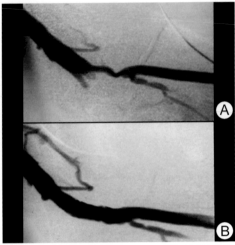

(A) Once thrombolysis performed evaluate venous outflow and angioplasty venous stenosis. (B) Then evaluate arterial end, and if resistant clot, sweep with occlusion/thrombectomy catheter.

Procedure

<u>Patient Position/Location</u>
- Perform in holding area or other monitored area

<u>Procedure Steps</u>
- Prep site close to arterial anastomosis, give anesthesia
- Needle directed towards venous anastomosis
- Grasp graft between thumb and forefinger of one hand
- Puncture graft with needle, there may be no blood return
- Try to aspirate to verify placement, no blood return probably try again
- Manually compress arterial and venous anastomosis
- Inject thrombolytic into graft
  - tPA 2 mg in 5-10 cc
  - Reteplase 3-5 mg in 5-10 cc
  - Heparin 2-3,000 units intravenously
- Wait 30-60 minutes (lyse and wait) or immediately start procedure in angiographic room (lyse and go)
- Evaluate venous outflow stenosis
- Evaluate venous outflow to the level of the right atrium
- Identify venous stenosis and treat per dialysis angioplasty chapter
- Evaluate arterial anastomosis
- If arterial end has resistant clot
  - Treat per chapter on dialysis thrombolysis
- When good angiographic result
  - Patient going to dialysis, exchange catheter for dialysis sheath
  - If patient not going to dialysis, remove catheter, hold **gentle** pressure

<u>Alternative Procedures/Therapies</u>
- Radiologic
  - Cross-catheter technique
  - Thrombectomy devices
- Surgical

o Thrombectomy
o Angiographic evaluation and angioplasty following thrombectomy

Post-Procedure
Things to Do
• Immediate dialysis with full anticoagulation
• Consider antiplatelet and anticoagulants
• Consider scheduled appointment in 3-4 months
Things to Avoid
• No tight dressings

Common Problems & Complications
Unable to Determine if Catheter within the Graft
• Avoid injecting in perigraft tissues
• Use cross-catheter technique, see chapter on dialysis thrombolysis
Bleeding from Previous Puncture Sites
• Manually compress
• Begin procedure as quickly as possible
• Angioplasty venous stenosis as quickly as possible
Unable to Thrombolyse Graft
• Reassess technique, use cross-catheter technique
• Possible infected thrombus-resistant to thrombolysis

Selected References
1. Falk A et al: Thrombolysis of clotted hemodialysis grafts with tissue-type plasminogen activator. JVIR 12: 305-11, 2001
2. Falk A et al: Reteplase in the treatment of thrombosed hemodialysis grafts. JVIR 12: 1257-62, 2001
3. Cynamon J et al: Hemodialysis graft declotting: Description of the "lyse and wait" technique. JVIR 10:96-8, 1999

Femoral Dialysis Catheter

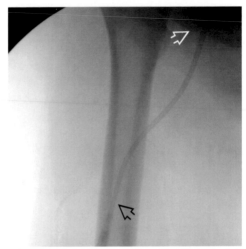

Permanent right femoral dialysis catheter. Note: Long tunnel extends laterally away from inguinal area. Proximal part of tunnel is made relatively deep. (White open arrow) shows site of skin nick for venipuncture. (Black open arrow) shows tunnel exit site.

Key Facts
- Make skin nick along Langer's lines
- Common femoral vein is medial to common femoral artery
- Use ultrasound for venipuncture when available
- Place extra stiff guide wire into IVC
- Make tunnel and tunnel exit deep
- Align sheath with wire and twist as advance in small increments

Pre-Procedure
Indications
- Renal failure requiring hemodialysis with SVC occlusion
- Infections and venous occlusions preventing placement of a catheter into neck and chest veins

Contraindications
- Infection at planned site
- Thrombosis of entry vein, iliac vein or IVC

Getting Started
- Things to Check
  - Bleeding history, INR, PTT, platelets
  - Previous catheter history
  - Previous and planned dialysis graft surgeries
  - Examine planned area of placement
    - Check for signs of previous surgeries or infections
  - Can check vein with ultrasound prior to prepping target area
    - Confirm venous patency and absence of DVT
- Equipment List
  - Temporary dialysis catheter or 45 to 55 cm permanent catheter

Femoral Dialysis Catheter

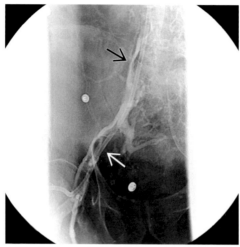

DVT of external iliac (white arrow) and common iliac (black arrow) veins due to right femoral dialysis catheter.

Procedure

Patient Position
- Supine

Choice of Vein
- Right femoral vein is better entry site because right iliac vein straighter and shorter than left

Target Site for Vein Entry
- Best site to enter is around junction of mid and lower thirds of femoral head
  - Ensures entry below inguinal ligament

Procedure Steps
- Make skin nick parallel to Langer's lines
  - Heals better and is easier to suture
- Use ultrasound to obtain access to vein and then place 0.035", Amplatz, extra stiff guidewire into IVC

Making Tunnel for "Permanent" Catheters
- Make tunnel at least 10 cm long and directed laterally
  - Decreases risk of infection
- Make tunnel and tunnel exit from venipuncture nick deep, as decreases risk of infection and easier to suture venipuncture nick

Placing Peel Away Sheath and Catheter
- Placing peel away sheath is the most dangerous part of procedure
  - Difficulty is large size of sheath and step-off between sheath and dilator, consider predilating with fascial dilators
  - Align sheath with wire and twist as advance in small increments
  - Once peel away component is in vein, resistance will decrease

Placing Catheter thru Peel Away Sheath
- Make sure that both lumens of catheter are clamped
- As dilator is coming out of peel away, pinch peel away sheath
- Prevents bleeding or air embolus
- Now advance catheter into sheath

Femoral Dialysis Catheter

- Check location of catheter tip under fluoroscopy
- Sometimes a glidewire will be needed to steer catheter into IVC
  - 0.035" angle tip glidewire is placed thru blue lumen and into IVC
- Sometimes a glidewire will be needed just to get catheter to go thru peel away sheath and into vein

Location for Catheter Tip
- Make sure notched side hole is pointed away from IVC wall

Test That a Dialysis Catheter Has "Good Flow"
- Desirable flow rate is greater than or equal to 300 cc/minute
- Use a 10 cc syringe to check flow rate
  - If you can pull back 10 cc in 2 seconds, that is equivalent to 300 cc/minute

Flushing and Securing Catheter
- Goal is to fill catheter with flush solution and to avoid backflow of blood into tip of catheter
- This is accomplished by clamping clamp while still flushing
- Most common mistake is to stop flushing and then clamp
  - Allows blood to flow into catheter tip

Temporary Dialysis Catheters
- Placed without a subcutaneous tunnel
  - Easier and faster to place than tunneled catheters
- Have firm, tapered tip for over-the-wire placement
- Do not have a cuff
- Typically are placed for short-time use in inpatients or for one time use in outpatients
- Higher infection rate than tunneled catheters
- Some nursing homes will not accept patients with nontunneled catheters

Permanent Dialysis Catheters
- Have soft tip which requires peel-away sheath for placement
- Have a cuff which requires tunnel for placement
  - Scar tissue forms around cuff and helps form barrier to infection and helps prevent dislodgement

Post-Procedure

Things to Do
- Observe for at least one hour or send to dialysis unit
- Monitor puncture site for bleeding and hematoma

Common Problems and Complications
- Infection is most common complication
- Hematoma in leg or pelvis
- IVC, iliac and femoral vein thrombosis

Selected References
1. Zaleski GX et al: Experience with tunneled femoral hemodialysis catheters. AJR 172: 493-6, 1999
2. Docktor BL et al: Radiologic placement of tunneled catheters: Rates of success and immediate complications in a large series. AJR 173:457-60, 1999
3. Abu-Yousef et al: Normal lower limb venous doppler phasicity: Is it cardiac or respiratory? AJR 169:1721-5, 1997

Jugular Dialysis Catheter

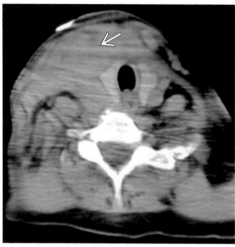

Right neck hematoma (white arrow) after attempted internal jugular vein puncture by palpation.

Key Facts
- Right internal jugular vein is best location for dialysis catheters
- Make skin nick along Langer's lines
- Use ultrasound and micropuncture needle for venipuncture
- Place extra stiff, guidewire into inferior vena cava (IVC)
- Make tunnel and tunnel exit deep
- Align sheath with wire and twist as advance in small increments
- Only insert peel away sheath to halfway point
- Pinch sheath with fingers to avoid air embolism
- Optimal tip location is upper right atrium (RA)

Pre-Procedure
Indications
- Renal failure requiring hemodialysis
- Plasmapheresis

Contraindications
- Infection at planned site
- Occlusion of superior vena cava (SVC)
- Occlusion of entry vein (relative contraindication)

Getting Started
- Things to Check
  - Previous catheter history
  - Previous and planned dialysis graft surgeries
  - Bleeding and anticoagulation history
  - Examine planned area of placement
    - Check for any signs of previous catheters, surgeries or infections and abundant collateral veins suggest subclavian and or jugular venous occlusion
  - Check if any previous venous ultrasound or venogram of target area
- Equipment List
  - A 19 cm catheter from tip to cuff is equivalent to 36 cm from tip to hub

Jugular Dialysis Catheter

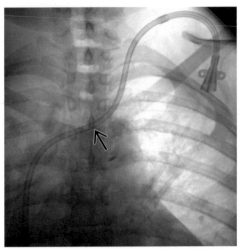

Left internal jugular vein tunneled dialysis catheter (arrow). Note: Left jugular catheters travel a longer distance to reach the right atrium than does a right sided catheter.

- o A 23 cm tip to cuff catheter is equivalent to 40 cm from tip to hub
- o Usually 36 or 40 cm catheters are placed from a right jugular or subclavian approach
- o Usually 40 or 45 cm catheters are placed from a left jugular or subclavian approach

Imaging Recommendations
- If multiple previous catheters, then check vein with ultrasound prior to prepping target area

Procedure

Patient Position/Location
- Supine
- Procedure table should be parallel to ground, not Trendelenburg

Right Internal Jugular Vein Puncture
- Make skin nick parallel to Langer's lines
  - o This heals better and is easier to suture
- Use a horizontal, anterior approach
- Advance 0.018" guidewire into SVC
- Place 5 French coaxial micropuncture dilator
- Exchange for 75 cm long, Amplatz extra stiff wire
- Advance extra stiff wire down into inferior vena cava (IVC)
  - o Be gentle
  - o Check monitor for arrhythmia
  - o If necessary, use hockey stick catheter to steer guide wire
  - o 40 cm Berenstein catheter works well to steer guide wire LAO projection throws right atrium off spine to show wire
- Now make tunnel

Making the Tunnel
- Easier to make tunnel now, since only 5 French dilator is in vein entry site
- Make tunnel so that crosses clavicle at or just lateral to midclavicular line

Jugular Dialysis Catheter

- Tunnel should extend from 3 cm caudal to clavicle up to site of skin nick for venipuncture
- Use 1% lidocaine to anesthetize tunnel tract
  - This also creates a plane to facilitate passage of tunneler
- Metal tunnelers are easier than plastic, be careful not to cut yourself
- Bend metal tunneler at right angle to facilitate exit at venipuncture site
- Jam catheter tightly onto tunneler
- If the patient has had previous catheters, then use a hemostat to open up tunnel tract and to get through scar tissue
- Make tunnel and tunnel exit from venipuncture nick deep, as this decreases risk of infection and makes it easier to suture venipuncture nick
- Key step is to push catheter as pull tunneler through venipuncture site
  - Prevents separation from tunneler

Sheath and Catheter
- Most dangerous part of procedure
- If large dilator passed too forcefully and wire kinks, dilator may pass through wall of SVC
- Align sheath with wire and twist as advance in small increments
- Guide wire and dilator should move freely relative to each other
- Only insert peel-away sheath to halfway point
  - Minimizes sheath kinking
- Make sure both ports on catheter are flushed and clamped
- Remove guide wire and sheath dilator
- Pinch sheath with fingers to avoid air embolism and advance catheter through sheath
- If catheter won't go through sheath, use glidewire through blue lumen
- Optimal tip location is upper right atrium (RA)
- Use syringe test to confirm function
- 10 ml blood aspirated in 2 seconds correlates to flow rate of 300 ml/min
- Flush both ports with heparinized saline, 100 units heparin/ml
- Suture catheter to skin with 3-0 monofilament nylon suture

Post-Procedure
Things to Do
- Observe for one hour or send to dialysis unit
- If any concern of pneumothorax, then obtain chest x-ray
- Chest x-ray is usually not needed if ultrasound used

Common Problems & Complications
- Pneumothorax
- SVC laceration
- Catheter, kink, thrombosis and infection
- Arrhythmia
- Jugular vein thrombosis and SVC thrombosis

Selected References
1. Trerotola SO et al: Tunneled infusion catheters: Increased incidence of symptomatic venous thrombosis after subclavian versus internal jugular venous access. RJ 217:89-93, 2000
2. Sasadeusz KJ et al: Tunneled jugular small-bore central catheters as an alternative to peripherally inserted central catheters for intermediate-term venous access in patients with hemodialysis and chronic renal insufficiency. RJ 213:303-6, 1999
3. Trerotola SO et al: Outcome of hemodialysis catheters placed via the right internal jugular vein by interventional radiologists. RJ 203:489-95, 1997

Recanalized Vein Catheter

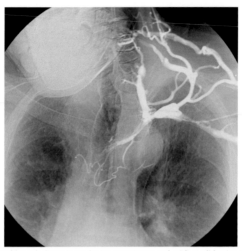

This left brachiocephalic vein occlusion was traversed with a glidewire and hockey stick tip catheter. Exchange for an extra stiff guidewire was made and the tract serially dilated prior to placement of a tunneled dialysis catheter.

Key Facts
- Dialysis catheters can usually be placed thru stenotic subclavian veins
- If traversable with a guidewire, an occluded subclavian vein can usually be recanalized with serial dilation or balloon angioplasty
- Dialysis catheters can be placed thru recanalized subclavian veins
- Reopening the subclavian vein for placement of a dialysis catheter spares other sites from catheter related stenosis or occlusion
- External jugular vein and other collateral veins can be used for catheter placement
  - However, these sites lead to increased procedure duration and difficulty

Pre-Procedure
Indications
- Renal failure requiring hemodialysis
Contraindications
- Infection at planned site
- Occlusion of superior vena cava (SVC)
Getting Started
- Things to Check
  - Previous catheter history and previous or planned dialysis graft surgeries
  - Bleeding and anticoagulation history
  - Examine planned area of placement
  - Check if any previous venous ultrasound or venogram of target area
    - Previous venograms are very helpful
- Equipment List
  - Micropuncture kit with 21-gauge needle, 0.018" wire and coaxial dilator
  - 0.035", angled-tip, stiff glidewire and a torque control device
  - Amplatz, extra stiff, 0.035" guidewire

Recanalized Vein Catheter

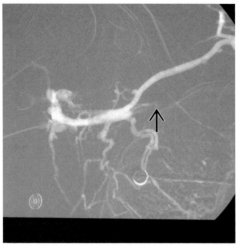

Right axillary vein and distal subclavian vein are occluded (black arrow) following previous subclavian catheter. Severe stenosis of SVC was also present. Lesions were traversed and balloon angioplasty done. Dialysis catheter was placed across the recanalized segment.

- Hockey-stick-tip catheter
- Amplatz, goose neck, loop snare is sometimes helpful
- Usually 36 or 40 cm catheters are placed from a right chest or neck approach
- Usually 40 or 45 cm catheters are placed from a left chest or neck approach

Procedure

Patient Position
- Supine

Axillary Vein Approach
- Obtain access to proximal axillary vein with ultrasound guidance
- Advance 0.018″ guidewire across subclavian stenosis and into SVC
- Place 5 French coaxial micropuncture dilator
- Exchange for 75 cm long, Amplatz extra stiff wire and place into IVC
- Serially dilate subclavian vein stenosis and place dialysis catheter

Upper Extremity Approach
- Obtain access to arm vein and place a long sheath
- Cross subclavian stenosis with hockey stick tip catheter and stiff glidewire
- Perform balloon angioplasty to dilate subclavian vein
  - Fix balloon securely at skin level so that it does not move when inflated
- For difficult cases it can be helpful to also obtain access to common femoral vein and to pull an exchange length guidewire with loop snare technique thru the femoral access
  - This "through and through" access makes it easier to advance angioplasty balloons across tight subclavian stenoses
- Use ultrasound and/or fluoroscopic guidance with indwelling guidewire to puncture proximal, ipsilateral axillary vein and place dialysis catheter

Recanalized Vein Catheter

Common Femoral Vein Approach
- Obtain access to right femoral vein and place a hockey tip catheter into a target vein e.g. a superficial, anterior collateral neck vein
- Evaluate site of catheter with ultrasound to determine if reachable with a needle without traversing a large or medium sized artery
- Catheter in vein serves as a target for fluoroscopically guided puncture with a 21-gauge needle
- After 0.018" guidewire is placed into SVC
  - Can reevaluate area with ultrasound to confirm medium or large arteries not traversed
- Dialysis catheter is then placed
- Suture catheter to skin with 3-0 monofilament nylon suture

Post-Procedure
Things to Do
- Observe for one hour or send to dialysis unit
- If any concern of pneumothorax, then obtain chest x-ray

Common Problems & Complications
- Pneumothorax
- Subclavian vein perforation
- SVC laceration
- Catheter, kink, thrombosis and infection
- Arrhythmia

Selected References
1. Funaki B et al: Radiologic placement of tunneled hemodialysis catheters in occluded neck, chest, or small thyrocervical collateral veins in central venous occlusion. Radiology 218: 471-476, 2001
2. Hagen P et al: Use of an amplatz goose neck snare as a target for collateral neck vein dialysis catheter placement. JVIR 12: 493-5, 2001
3. Forauer AR et al: Placement of hemodialysis catheters through dilated external jugular and collateral veins in patients with internal jugular vein occlusions. AJR 174:361-2, 2000

Subclavian Dialysis Catheter

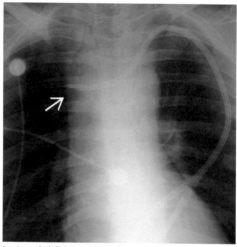

Left subclavian tunneled dialysis catheter (arrow) is too short and has tipped upward within superior vena cava. Catheter functioned poorly and had to be exchanged. Longer catheters are typically needed on left side in comparison with right.

Key Facts
- Use ultrasound and micropuncture needle for venipuncture
- Place extra stiff, guidewire into IVC
- Align sheath with wire and twist as advance in small increments
- Pinch sheath with fingers to avoid air embolism
- Optimal tip location is upper to mid right atrium (RA)
- For a more detailed discussion of subclavian vein puncture, please see chapter devoted to that topic
- Right jugular vein approach is preferred, subclavian vein is used as an alternative

Pre-Procedure
Indications
- Renal failure requiring hemodialysis
- Plasmapheresis

Contraindications
- Infection at planned site
- Occlusion of entry vein or superior vena cava (SVC)

Getting Started
- Things to Check
  - Previous catheter history
  - Previous and planned dialysis graft surgeries
  - Bleeding and anticoagulation history
  - Examine planned area of placement
    - Check for signs of previous catheters, surgeries or infections
    - Abundant collateral veins suggest subclavian and/or jugular occlusion
  - Check if any previous ultrasound or venogram of target area
- Equipment List
  - A 19 cm catheter tip to cuff is equivalent to 36 cm from tip to hub

Subclavian Dialysis Catheter

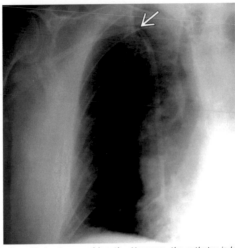

Right subclavian catheter is a good length. However, the catheter is kinked (white arrow) at the junction of subclavian and brachiocephalic veins. This is a common site for catheter to kink.

- o A 23 cm tip to cuff catheter is equivalent to 40 cm from tip to hub
- o Usually 36 or 40 cm catheters placed with right subclavian approach
- o Usually 40 or 45 cm catheters placed with left subclavian approach

Imaging Recommendations
- If has had previous subclavian catheters, then check vein with ultrasound prior to prepping target area

Procedure
Patient Position
- Supine with procedure table parallel to ground

Subclavian Vein Puncture
- Make skin nick parallel to Langer's lines as this heals better
- Ultrasound guided puncture is most common technique
  - o Other options for guidance are venography or palpation of anatomical landmarks
- Ultrasound guided punctures are typically located more laterally than landmark guided puncture
- Slight jabbing motion as needle enters vein facilitates single wall entry
  - o Advance 0.018" guidewire into SVC
- Place 5 French coaxial micropuncture dilator
- Exchange for 75 cm long, Amplatz extra stiff wire and gently advance down into inferior vena cava (IVC)
  - o If necessary, use 40 cm, hockey stick tip catheter to steer guidewire

Making the Tunnel
- In large patients vein is located deep and puncture tract is long enough to serve as "tunnel" for placement of cuff
- In smaller patients, a 3 to 7 cm long tunnel is directed caudally
- Use 1% lidocaine to anesthetize tunnel tract
- Bend metal tunneler at right angle to facilitate exit at venipuncture site

Subclavian Dialysis Catheter

- Make tunnel and tunnel exit from venipuncture nick deep, as this decreases risk of infection and makes it easier to suture venipuncture nick
- Jam catheter tightly onto tunneler and push catheter as pull tunneler through venipuncture site as this prevents separation from tunneler

<u>Sheath and Catheter</u>
- Only insert peel away sheath to halfway point to minimize sheath kinking
- There are several keys to completing this part of procedure safely
  - o Use an Amplatz, extra stiff guidewire placed down into IVC
  - o Align sheath with wire and twist as advance in small increments
  - o Gently pull wire back and forth slightly as sheath advanced
    - Guidewire and dilator should move freely relative to each other
    - Dilator moving freely relative to wire, indicates wire not kinked
- Main site of resistance is when sheath step-off relative to sheath dilator contacts fascial tissue around vein
- Once sheath component is in vein, resistance will decrease
- Remove guidewire and sheath dilator
- Pinch sheath to avoid air embolism
- Place blue hub laterally with right sided approach as this usually orients catheter so that sideholes go to a favorable location in right atrium
- Advance catheter through sheath
- If catheter won't go through sheath, use glidewire through blue lumen
- Optimal tip location is upper to mid right RA
- Flush both ports with heparinized saline, 100 units heparin/ml
- Suture catheter to skin with 3-0 monofilament nylon suture

Post-Procedure
- Observe for at least one hour or send to dialysis unit
- If any concern of pneumothorax, then view lung apex with fluoroscopy
  - o Place chest tube if large, symptomatic pneumothorax present
- If clinical symptoms suggest pneumothorax, yet none seen on fluoroscopy then obtain upright AP expiration and inspiration CXR
  - o Keep patient in department until have viewed CXR

Common Problems & Complications
- Difficulty advancing dilators may occur with steep approach angle
- Pneumothorax is rare with ultrasound guidance
  - o However, in large patients, the subclavian vein can be difficult to see with ultrasound
- Catheter, kink, thrombosis and infection
- Arterial puncture may lead to hematoma or arteriovenous fistula
- Arrhythmia
- SVC laceration
- Subclavian vein stenosis or occlusion which can lead to arm swelling or ipsilateral dialysis graft poor function
  - o Occurs in a moderate number of patients
  - o Much more common than catheter related jugular vein thrombosis

Selected References
1. Funaki B et al: Radiologic placement of tunneled hemodialysis catheters in occluded neck, chest, or small thyrocervical collateral veins in central venous occlusion. Radiology 218:471-6, 2001
2. Trerotola S et al: Tunneled infusion catheters: Increased incidence of symptomatic venous thrombosis after subclavian versus internal jugular venous access. Radiology 217:89-93, 2000
3. Muhm M et al: Supraclavicular approach to the subclavian/innominate vein for large-bore central venous catheters. Am J of Kidney Dis 30:802-8, 1997

Translumbar Dialysis Catheter

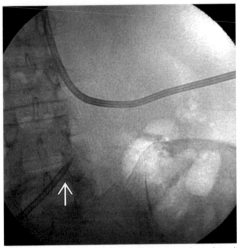

Indwelling femoral vein temporary dialysis catheter (arrow) used to obtain inferior vena cavagram. Cavagram used as a guide for translumbar IVC puncture. Translumbar IVC catheter is also seen.

Key Facts
- Translumbar dialysis catheter placement involves fluoroscopic guided puncture of inferior vena cava (IVC)
- Patients typically have central venous occlusions which prevent placement of a subclavian or jugular dialysis catheter

Pre-Procedure
Indications
- Renal failure requiring hemodialysis with central venous occlusions which prevent placement of a subclavian or jugular dialysis catheter e.g. SVC occlusion

Contraindications
- Infection at planned site
- Thrombosis of IVC

Getting Started
- Things to Check
  o Bleeding history, INR, PTT, platelets and hemoglobin
  o Previous catheter history
  o Previous and planned dialysis graft surgeries
  o Examine planned area of placement
  o Consider prophylactic antibiotics such as Ancef or vancomycin
- Equipment List
  o Long, 18-gauge (G) needle
  o 145 cm long, 3 mm J tip guidewire and 40 cm hockey-stick-tip catheter
  o 75 cm Amplatz, extra stiff guidewire
  o 5, 7, 9, 11 French dilators
  o 13.5 French, 45 to 60 cm long dialysis catheter with a cuff
  o 0.035", angled tip, stiff glidewire

Translumbar Dialysis Catheter

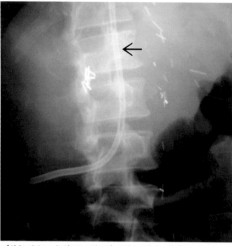

Key feature of this picture is that patient's right side is slightly elevated leading to an oblique image. Slight elevation of the patient's right side facilitates subcutaneous tunneling of the catheter. (Arrow) points to catheter in IVC.

- May need an extra long, e.g. 30 cm, peel away sheath for large patients

Procedure
Patient Position
- Supine initially if intend to place a 5 French sheath into femoral vein
  - Contrast is injected thru it or a pigtail catheter can be placed into IVC
  - This makes IVC puncture easier and faster
- Prone for translumbar puncture of IVC
  - Approximately 15 degrees elevation of patient's right side facilitates later tunneling out towards midaxillary line
Target Site for Vein Entry
- Patients will often have an indwelling temporary femoral catheter
  - If not, then place a sheath and/or a pigtail catheter
- Inject contrast to opacify IVC and can obtain a "roadmap"
  - Can also use a catheter placed into IVC as a target for puncture
- Skin entry site is 8-10 cm lateral to midline and 2 cm above iliac crest
- Best site to enter infrarenal IVC is just below level of L3 pedicle
- Orient image intensifier along planned needle path so that needle hub will be superimposed over tip
- Put IVC target into center of field of view
- Magnify as much as possible
- 22 G spinal needle is placed along planned path to give local anesthetic
- Advance long, 18 G needle into IVC followed by 3 mm J tip guidewire
- Exchange needle for 5 French hockey-stick-tip catheter and place into IVC
- Place guidewire 1 cm into right atrium, then clamp wire where exits catheter with a hemostat
  - Subtract catheter length protruding from skin to determine length of wire inside patient and thus how long of a catheter is needed

Translumbar Dialysis Catheter

Making Tunnel
- Make tunnel out to midaxillary line
- Keep tunnel cephalad to iliac crest so will not later be compressed when patient is supine
- Pull catheter thru tunnel

Placing Peel-Away Sheath and Catheter
- Dilate tract and place peel-away sheath into IVC
  - May need a long peel-away sheath
  - Align sheath with wire and twist as advance in small increments
  - Once peel-away component is in vein, resistance will decrease
  - Only advance a short distance into IVC to prevent kinking of sheath

Placing Catheter thru Peel-Away Sheath
- Place 0.035", angled-tip, stiff glidewire thru blue lumen of dialysis catheter
- As dilator is coming out of peel away, pinch peel away sheath
  - Prevents bleeding or air embolus
- Now advance catheter thru sheath into IVC
- Check location of catheter tip under fluoroscopy

Catheter Tip Location
- Make sure notched sidehole is pointed away from IVC wall
- Place distal tip of catheter approximately 1 cm into right atrium

Test that a Dialysis Catheter has "Good Flow"
- Desirable flow rate is greater than or equal to 300 cc/minute
  - Use a 10 cc syringe to check flow rate
  - If you can pull back 10 cc in 2 seconds, that is equivalent to 300 cc/minute
- Suture catheter to skin with 3-0 monofilament nylon

Post-Procedure

Things to Do
- Observe for at least 6 hours while monitor blood pressure and pulse
- Do not administer heparin for at least 24 hours

Common Problems and Complications
- Pain in back and/or right leg
- Infection
- Injury to right ureter
- Hematoma in psoas muscle
- Retroperitoneal hemorrhage requiring blood transfusion
  - If suspect bleeding, stabilize patient, measure hemoglobin and obtain a CT scan of abdomen and pelvis
- Inadvertent catheter dislodgement
- IVC thrombosis

Selected References
1. Patel NH: Percutaneous translumbar placement of a Hickman catheter into the azygous vein. AJR 175: 1302-4, 2000
2. Rajan DL et al: Translumbar placement of inferior vena cava catheters: A solution for challenging hemodialysis access. Radiographics 18: 115-67, 1998
3. Bennett JD et al: Percutaneous inferior vena caval approach for long-term central venous access. JVIR 8:851-5, 1997

PocketRadiologist™
Interventional
Top 100 Procedures

ARTERIAL

Abdominal Aortogram

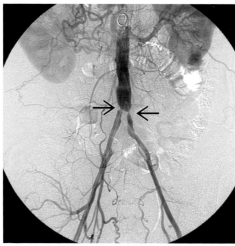

Stenosis of bilateral common iliac artery (CIA) origins (arrows). These lesions were successfully treated with simultaneous deployment of bilateral CIA origin, balloon expandable stents.

Key Facts
- Peripheral vascular disease (PVD) is most common indication
- Goal is to determine cause of symptoms as well as potential percutaneous and surgical treatment options
- Routine abdominal aortogram typically includes abdominal aorta, main renal arteries and iliac arteries

Pre-Procedure
Indications
- PVD
- Mesenteric ischemia
- Abdominal aortic aneurysm (AAA)
- Renal artery stenosis and renal transplant donor evaluation

Contraindications
- Uncorrectable bleeding diathesis
- Bilateral common femoral artery (CFA) occlusions
  - Procedure can still be done from arm
- Moderate renal failure is relative contraindication
  - Hydrate
  - Consider other nephroprotective agents
  - Minimize contrast load

Getting Started
- Things to Check
  - Check if patient on heparin or Coumadin
  - Check creatinine, platelets and INR
  - Check which leg is more symptomatic
    - Puncture other side
  - Check history previous vascular surgery
    - Try to avoid puncture of surgical graft unless no other good option
  - Check femoral pulses

Abdominal Aortogram

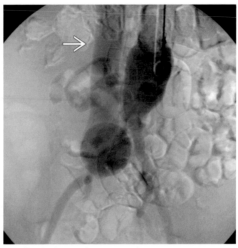

Arteriovenous fistula *from right common iliac artery aneurysm to inferior vena cava which is dilated (arrow) due to high flow state.*

- Equipment List
  - 4 or 5 French sheath
  - 65 cm long, 4 or 5 French pigtail, tennis racquet or Omni Flush catheter

Procedure
<u>Patient Position</u>
- Supine

<u>Equipment Preparation</u>
- Flush catheters, wires and sheath

<u>Procedure Steps</u>
- Place a 5 French sheath in CFA
- Place a pigtail or similar multi-side-hole catheter in aorta just distal to expected location of renal arteries
- Check that pigtail or tennis racquet catheter is "fully opened" within abdominal aorta
  - Distal catheter loop will appear constricted if within a stenosis
- Do a hand injection of contrast to confirm catheter is not within a dissection and to check catheter position relative to renal arteries
- Pigtail catheters usually lead to a significant upward reflux of contrast
  - Do not place above renal arteries for routine evaluation of PVD because large amount contrast may reflux upward and go into celiac trunk and SMA

<u>Routine View</u>
- A single posteroanterior (PA) view is usually adequate for evaluation of PVD
- Usual injection rate is 15 cc per second for a total of 30 cc contrast (15/ 30) or 20/40
- Decreasing source to image distance (SID) by elevating table and lowering image intensifier (II) will increase field of view size

Abdominal Aortogram

Lateral View
- Lateral view important for evaluation of mesenteric ischemia and AAA
  - Place catheter above celiac trunk
  - Check for occlusion of celiac trunk and superior mesenteric artery
  - Check relationship of celiac artery, SMA, renal arteries and IMA to AAA

Oblique View
- Oblique views are helpful for evaluation of renal artery stenosis
  - Renal artery ostium is most common site of severe stenosis
- Oblique views also helpful for evaluation of abdominal aorta stenoses
  - If stenosis seen on routine PA view, then get an oblique and/or lateral view
- Oblique roadmap angiography is helpful for selective catheterization of celiac trunk, SMA and inferior mesenteric artery (IMA)

Inferior Mesenteric Artery
- Contrast is heavier than blood and tends to layer posteriorly in abdominal aorta
- IMA has a relatively anterior origin from abdominal aorta and may not opacify when catheter is in proximal abdominal aorta
- Placement of pigtail or tennis racquet catheter in distal abdominal aorta facilitates flush arteriography opacification of IMA

Left Arm Approach
- Use a 100 cm long pigtail catheter
- 0.035" angled-tip glidewire is passed from left brachial artery down into descending thoracic aorta (DTA)
  - If wire repeatedly goes into subclavian artery side branches, then a 3 mm J tip or Rosen guidewire may be used
  - LAO view helps to open up aortic arch to facilitate passage of wire into DTA
  - Pigtail catheter is usually adequate for steering wire into DTA
  - In some patients will need to use hockey-tip-type catheter

Removal of Pigtail Catheter
- Catheter is typically removed over a guidewire
- Guidewire straightens tip of pigtail catheter so that it is less likely to catch on atherosclerotic plaque
- It is especially important to "pull over a guidewire" when the catheter will be pulled across a stent

Post-Procedure

Things to Do
- Obtain hemostasis, bed rest for 6 hours, monitor puncture site and pulses

Common Problems & Complications

Complications
- Inadequate opacification of arteries in symptomatic region
- Puncture site complications such as dissection and hematoma
- Iliac or femoral artery thrombosis

Selected References
1. Hartnell G et al: MR angiography compared with digital subtraction angiography. AJR 175:1188-9, 2000
2. Gates J et al: Optimized diagnostic angiography in high-risk patients with severe peripheral vascular disease. Radiographics 20:121-33, 2000
3. Alson MD et al: Pedal Arterial Imaging. JVIR 8:9-18, 1997

Brachial Artery Puncture

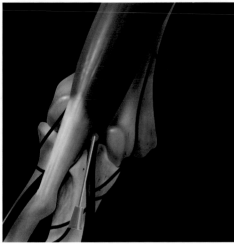

Left brachial artery is punctured just proximal to the antecubital region with ultrasound guidance.

Key Facts
- Left brachial artery is a common entry site for angiography procedures

Pre-Procedure
Indications
- Angiography when both iliofemoral arteries severely diseased or occluded
- Common femoral artery region infection or recent surgical graft

Contraindications
- Uncorrectable bleeding diathesis
- Known occlusion of brachial artery

Getting Started
- Things to Check
  - Check brachial, radial and ulnar pulses in arm
    - Document to serve as baseline
  - Left arm is used because only cross vertebral artery on way to aortic arch
    - On right side cross right vertebral and carotid ostia as well as left carotid and left subclavian
- Equipment List
  - Micropuncture kit with a 21-gauge needle
  - 4 to 6 French sheath with short length wire that comes in sheath kit
  - 3 mm J tip guidewire or a Rosen, 1.5 mm J tip guidewire
  - Heparin at a concentration of 1,000 units per cc
  - Nitroglycerin (NTG) in a concentration of 100 micrograms per cc
  - Heparinized saline flush system for sidearm of sheath
    - 2000 units heparin in 1 liter 0.9 NS
    - Pressure bag should be pumped to 300 mm Hg

Procedure
Ultrasound
- Enables access with lack of a palpable pulse

Brachial Artery Puncture

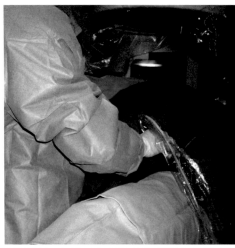

Setup for brachial artery puncture is same as for PICC line with arm extended at elbow. Tourniquet in axilla makes brachial veins taut to help fix position of brachial artery. Physician is holding ultrasound transducer over left brachial artery.

- Decreases pain and spasm by usually enabling access on first needle stick
- Allows direct visualization of needle being placed into artery
- Reduces risk of brachial vein arteriovenous fistula
- Enables front walling of artery reliably and decreases risk of bleeding if thrombolysis is done
- With U/S, artery is pulsatile and noncompressible
  - Vein is nonpulsatile and compressible
- Transducer is placed transverse relative to brachial artery
  - Decrease field of view depth as much as possible to magnify size of artery
  - Bigger target easier to hit
- Put artery in center of transducer field of view
  - Then put needle along center of transducer
  - Maintaining this alignment will facilitate arterial entry
- Try to visualize needle from skin entry down to artery
  - Works better than trying to find needle after already advanced inward
  - Needle tip is echogenic
  - Turning down 2D gain will increase visibility of tip
- Try to puncture center of artery
  - Better for guidewire advancement than when side of artery is punctured
- Blood return is observed and guidewire is advanced into vessel

Typical Sequence of Steps
- Prep arm like for a PICC line and put tourniquet in axilla
  - Distends brachial veins which help hold brachial artery in place
  - Without tourniquet, artery has tendency to "wiggle" away from needle
- Typical entry site is distal brachial artery just above antecubital crease
  - U/S used to determine location of brachial artery bifurcation
  - 2% lidocaine is given for local anesthetic
  - Scalpel is used to make small nick in skin

Brachial Artery Puncture

- o 21-gauge needle is guided into artery by ultrasound
- 0.018" guidewire is advanced thru needle
- 5 French micropuncture dilator is placed and wire is upsized to 0.035"
- Usually a 4 or 5 French sheath is then placed
  - o 6 French is maximum sheath size in average size vessels
- Pulsatile flow in sheath helps confirm intraluminal
  - o Contrast can be injected thru inner part of coaxial dilator to confirm
- If systemic blood pressure normal or high, inject 100 to 200 micrograms NTG thru sheath
  - o Decreases spasm and risk of perisheath thrombosis
- Also inject 2,000 units of heparin thru sheath sidearm
  - o More heparin can be given if procedure is prolonged
- 3 mm J and Rosen guidewires are helpful as they tend to stay in main vessel lumen and avoid side branches

Brachial versus Axillary Approach
- Brachial artery is easier to compress
- If pseudoaneurysm occurs, brachial site is easier to treat
- Bleeding due to axillary puncture may compress brachial plexus and extend thru axilla into chest wall
- Brachial artery puncture tends to be more comfortable for patient because elbow is extended
  - o Unlike position for axillary approach where elbow is flexed and arm abducted
- Advantage of axillary puncture is closer to iliac and femoral circulations which facilitates angioplasty and stenting

Post-Procedure
Things to Do
- Obtain hemostasis and monitor patient

Common Problems and Complications
- Brachial artery spasm
  - o 50 to 200 micrograms NTG boluses thru sheath can be helpful
- Brachial artery dissection
- Hematoma can occur as brachial artery difficult to compress due to its tendency to "wiggle" away when palpated
  - o Important to try to feel pulse when compressing
  - o Helps insure compression applied effectively over site of arterial entry
- Brachial artery hematomas can compress median nerve
  - o Vascular surgery should be consulted in event that may require surgical evacuation
  - o Most brachial artery hematomas are small and will resolve spontaneously
- Pseudoaneurysm and arteriovenous fistula

Selected References
1. Morin ME et al: Carotid artery: Percutaneous transbrachial selective arteriography with a 4-F catheter. Radiology 171:868-70, 1989
2. Smith DC et al: Medial Brachial fascial compartment syndrome: Anatomic basis of neuropathy after transaxillary arteriography. Radiology 173:149-54, 1989
3. Lipchick EO et al: Percutaneous brachial artery catheterization. Radiology 160:842-3, 1986

Lower GI Bleeding

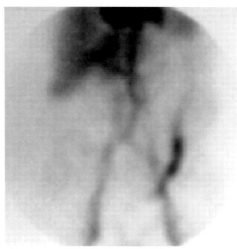

Red blood scan localizes site of bleeding, facilitates angiographic evaluation.

Key Facts
- Procedure definition: Evaluation /therapy of lower GI bleeding
- Clinical setting triggering procedure: Patient with blood per rectum
- Best procedure approach: Mesenteric angiogram-SMA, IMA, celiac
- Most feared complications: Ischemic bowel from therapy
- Expected outcome: Localization and treatment of lower GI bleed

Pre-Procedure
<u>Indications</u>
- Bright red bleeding per rectum or melanotic stools
- Hemodynamic instability
<u>Contraindications</u>
- Anaphylaxis to contrast agents
- Nuclear medicine scan not demonstrating active bleeding
<u>Getting Started</u>
- Things to Check
  - o Patient resuscitated, large caliber IV access, blood products
  - o Foley catheter –prevent bladder contrast from obscuring pelvis
  - o NG tube –verify bleeding from the lower track
  - o Sigmoidoscopy – avoid angiogram for hemorrhoidal bleeding
  - o Nuclear medicine scan if not massive continuous bleeding
- Equipment List
  - o Needle, 5 Fr dilator, 5 Fr sheath, hydrophilic wire
  - o Visceral catheter
    - ▪ Hook catheter, Cobra, Simmons, Rosch inferior mesenteric, etc.
  - o Embolization materials
    - ▪ Microcatheters, microwires, microcoils
  - o Vasopressin, Glucagon, conscious sedation

Procedure
<u>Patient Position/Location</u>
- Supine, standard angiographic approach

Lower GI Bleeding

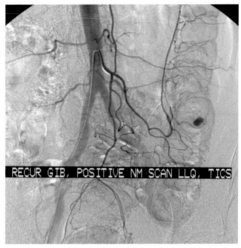

RECUR GIB, POSITIVE NM SCAN LLQ, TICS

Guided by the nuclear medicine study that demonstrated the bleeding on the left, inferior mesenteric artery injection demonstrates the bleeding site.

Procedure Steps
- Arteriographic puncture, placement of sheath
- Do not perform abdominal arteriogram – waste of contrast in most cases
- RBC study positive, study visceral vessel likely supplying bleeding site
- No nuclear medicine study, start with superior mesenteric angiogram (SMA), will evaluate the most bowel
- If unable to image the entire abdomen, then first run imaging right lower quadrant, second run imaging rest of SMA distribution
- No bleeding on the SMA injection(s), catheterize inferior mesenteric artery (IMA), may need two runs to cover IMA supplied bowel, visualize rectum
- No bleeding identified from IMA, celiac axis is selected and studied
- If bleeding site is found, make diagnosis of cause of bleeding
- Etiologies: Diverticular bleed, angiodysplasia, biopsy, AVM, varices, tumor, vasculitis, inflammatory bowel disease, Meckel's diverticulum, etc.
- Decision regarding therapy
  - Embolization
    - Localized lower GI bleed can be treated with embolization
    - Very selective catheterization, arcades proximal to vasa recta
    - Proximal embolization may result in ischemia
    - Microcoils preferred because of controllable placement
    - Gelfoam can be used but is less controllable
  - Vasopressin
    - Originally standard treatment, now used when subselective catheterization not possible, or diffuse process
    - Place catheter proximal visceral vessel
    - Infuse 0.2 U/min for 20 minutes then re-angiogram
    - Bleeding stopped, infusion continues 12-24 hours, patient in ICU
    - Bleeding continues, increase to 0.3-0.4 U/min, not >0.4 U/min
    - Taper by 0.1 U every 6 hours until infusing saline for 6 hours

Alternative Procedures/Therapies
- Surgical

- o Exploratory laparotomy and bowel resection high mortality up to 50% in acute bleeding, difficult to know where bleeding originates
- Endoscopy
  - o Usually not very helpful, difficult to visualize colon because of blood

Post-Procedure
Things to Do
- Post embolization, watch for evidence of bowel ischemia
- With vasopressin infusion watch for bowel ischemia, angina, dysrhythmias, fluid retention, complications of prolonged catheterization

Things to Avoid
- Enemas, laxatives, keep bowel at rest for a few days

Common Problems & Complications
Problems
- Difficulty catheterizing visceral vessels
  - o May be stenosis of vessel, do lateral aortogram to evaluate
- No bleeding found
  - o Patient stable hemodynamically, usually stop
  - o Patient still bleeding, consider unusual causes, aortoenteric fistula, iliac enteric fistula; restudy SMA
- Bleeding not found but then recurs
  - o Nuclear medicine scan to determine site restudy with angiography

Complications
- Injury to mesenteric vascular system from catheterization
- Bowel ischemia from embolization or vasopressin
- Ischemia in other sites (coronary, extremities, etc.) vasopressin

Selected References
1. Bandi R et al: Superselective arterial embolization for the treatment of lower gastrointestinal hemorrhage. JVIR 12:1399-1405, 2001
2. Lefkovitz Z et al: Radiology in the diagnosis and therapy of gastrointestinal bleeding. Gastroenterol Clin N Am 29:489-512, 2000
3. McKusick M: Interventional radiology for the control and prevention bleeding. Gastrointest Endosc Clin N Am 9:311-29, 1999

Hepatic Chemoembolization

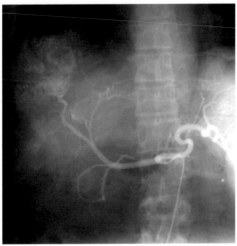

Selective injection into celiac axis. Hypervascular mass in right lobe with enlarged feeding artery, findings typical of hepatocellular carcinoma.

Key Facts
- Procedure synonyms: HACE
- Procedure definition: Treatment of hepatic malignancies with regional, catheter – directed chemotherapy
- Clinical setting triggering procedure: Primary or metastatic hepatic malignancies, patient not a surgical candidate
- Most feared complications: Hepatic necrosis, hepatic failure
- Expected outcome: Palliation; improved quality of life, decreased pain, constitutional symptoms; increased life expectancy; may allow liver transplant or hepatectomy

Pre-Procedure
Indications
- Hepatocellular carcinoma
- Hypervascular metastases: Carcinoid, islet cell, ocular melanoma
- Metastatic colorectal adenocarcinoma

Contraindications
- Severe liver failure, biliary obstruction
  - High risk patients: 50% of liver replaced by tumor, severe hepatic insufficiency LDH>425 IU/L, AST >100 IU/L, total bilirubin>2 mg/dl, encephalopathy or jaundice

Relative Contraindications
- Complete portal vein occlusion, extrahepatic metastatic disease, renal insufficiency, cardiac disease, severe thrombocytopenia

Getting Started
- Things to Check
  - Verification of pathology, previous imaging studies
  - Coagulation evaluation, creatinine, liver function tests, tumor markers (AFP, CEA, etc.), status of portal vein
  - Overnight fasting, Foley catheter, hydration (NS 200-300 cc/hr)
- Equipment List

Hepatic Chemoembolization

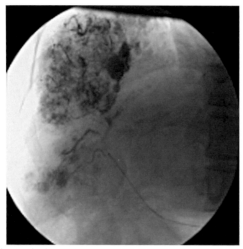

Post embolization (without contrast injection), density of the tumor is due to Ethiodol. Microcatheter seen in branch of right hepatic artery supplying tumor. Note second focal area of tumor inferior to main tumor.

- o 5 Fr sheath, Terumo glidewire
- o Selective visceral catheters- visceral hook, Cobra, Simmons
- o Microcatheters, microwires
- o Embolization material
  - ▪ Particles: PVA 300-500 μ, Biospheres 300-500 μ or 500-700 μ; Gelfoam, Ethiodol
  - ▪ Avoid coils
- o Chemotherapeutic agents, depends on malignancy
  - ▪ Commonly Mitomycin C, Doxorubicin, Cisplatin
  - ▪ Syringes 20 cc, 5 cc, 3 cc, 1 cc, 3-way stopcock
- o Medications
  - ▪ Antibiotics – Ancef and Flagyl
  - ▪ Analgesics – PCA
  - ▪ Antiemetics – Zofran, Decadron, Benadryl
- o Goggles or other eye protection when using chemotherapeutic agents

Procedure

Patient Position/Location
- • Supine, good angiographic visualization required

Equipment Preparation
- • Mix chemotherapeutic drugs with Ethiodol, and particles in large syringe with 3-way stopcock

Procedure Steps
- • Catheterize femoral artery, placement of sheath
- • Celiac arteriogram –variant hepatic artery anatomy, visualize portal vein
- • SMA angiogram –hepatic artery anomalies (replaced right hepatic artery), portal flow
- • If portal vein occluded, may still embolize but cautiously, only small areas
- • Selectively catheterize the hepatic artery branches supplying tumor
- • Subselectively catheterize as necessary

Hepatic Chemoembolization

- Embolize with mixture of chemotherapeutic agents, Ethiodol, and particles
- Watch for reflux of material into non-target vessels
- Spot film of liver evaluate distribution of embolization material, follow-up angiogram

Alternative Procedures/Therapies
- Radiologic
  - o Percutaneous ethanol, radiofrequency ablation
- Surgical
  - o Partial hepatectomy, orthotopic liver transplantation

Post-Procedure

Things to Do
- Hydration – NS 3L/24 hours (125 cc/hr), IV antibiotics, Zofran and Decadron q 8 hrs for 2 days, narcotics (PCA), NSAIDs, Compazine
- Discharge when able to eat, pain controlled on oral meds, Cipro 500 mg bid x 5 days, repeat labs 3-4 weeks, repeat procedure as necessary every 4-6 weeks
- Patient to be alert for fever, chills, increasing pain, increasing jaundice, increasing nausea/vomiting

Things to Avoid
- Patient should avoid excessive consumption of Tylenol, alcohol, protein

Common Problems & Complications

Problems
- Post-embolization syndrome is common
  - o Fever, abdominal pain, nausea
  - o IV hydration, antiemetics, PCA pump, antipyretics

Complications
- Severe
  - o Hepatic infarction, abscess, hepatic failure, tumor rupture
  - o Non-target embolization - gallbladder, stomach, small bowel
  - o Death
- Other complications
  - o Development of collaterals with continued blood supply to tumor, requires repeat embolization

Selected References
1. Sullivan KL et al: Hepatic artery chemoembolization. Semin Oncol 29:145-51, 2002
2. Leyendecker JR et al: Minimally invasive techniques for treatment of liver tumors. Semin Liver Dis 21:283-91, 2001
3. Yao KA et al: Indications and results of liver resection and hepatic chemoembolization for metastatic gastrointestinal neuroendocrine tumors. Surgery 130:677-82, 2001

Iliac Artery Angioplasty

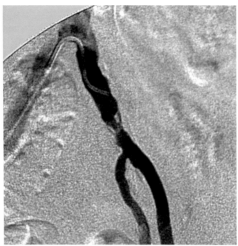

Complex, eccentric, focal stenosis of distal left common iliac artery. Note: Proximity of lesion to left internal iliac artery.

Key Facts
- Use exchange length, extra stiff guidewires
- Carefully choose balloon size and position

Pre-Procedure
Indications
- Symptomatic iliac artery stenosis amenable to percutaneous techniques
- To improve inflow to an ipsilateral e.g. femoral-popliteal bypass graft

Contraindications
- Uncorrectable bleeding diathesis
- Adjacent aneurysm

Getting Started
- Things to Check
  - Bleeding history, platelets, PT, PTT, INR, creatinine
  - Obtain a history and physical exam with emphasis on vascular disease
  - Check femoral, popliteal and foot pulses and/or Doppler signals
  - Administer aspirin
  - Hydration, especially if patient has marginal renal function
- Equipment List
  - 0.035" angled-tip glidewire for crossing lesion
  - 65 cm long hockey tip catheter for crossing lesion
  - 0.035" Amplatz extra stiff, exchange length guidewire
  - 6 to 8 French sheaths for balloon angioplasty and stenting
  - Angioplasty balloon(s) and stent(s)

Procedure
Patient Position
- Supine with both groins prepped

Procedure Steps
- Obtain diagnostic arteriogram with PA and bilateral oblique views of pelvis

Iliac Artery Angioplasty

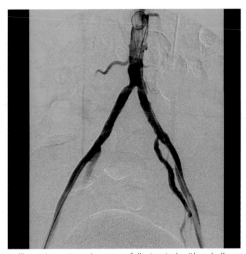

Left common iliac artery stenosis successfully treated with a balloon expandable stent dilated to 8 mm. Stent placed from ipsilateral femoral approach. Note: Left internal iliac artery remains intact.

- If uncertain of stenosis severity, intravascular pressures can be measured
- Do not need pressure measurement when stenosis is obviously severe
- Make decision on how will approach lesion, e.g. from ipsilateral or contralateral common femoral artery (I-CFA or C-CFA)
- In general, it is easier to work from I-CFA
  - Disadvantage is that often requires additional arterial puncture

Evaluation of Lesion
- Favorable findings are short segment, concentric stenosis
- Unfavorable findings are long segment, eccentric stenosis or occlusion in narrow diameter vessel, adjacent to important side branch, in patient with outflow disease who continues to smoke tobacco
- Long stenoses and occlusions are usually treated with stents or surgery
- Sites of failed angioplasty are usually treated with stents

Femoral Artery Access
- I-CFA is often pulseless
- Can puncture pulseless artery with ultrasound guidance
  - If access already obtained from C-CFA, a catheter in aorta can be used for roadmapping as guide to femoral puncture

Crossing Lesion
- Important to remain in true lumen
- From I-CFA, lesion can be crossed with a 0.035" angled tip glidewire and a hockey tip catheter with a magnified view roadmap for guidance
- If catheter is occlusive or nearly occlusive, then give heparin
- Exchange catheter for an Amplatz, extra stiff, exchange length guidewire
  - Will provide increased support for balloons and stents
- Based on diagnostic arteriogram, choose balloon size
- Remove air from angioplasty balloon and prepare insufflator

Balloon Angioplasty
- Typical balloon sizes for common iliac artery are 7-10 mm
- Typical balloon sizes for external iliac artery are 5-8 mm

Iliac Artery Angioplasty

Ostial Common Iliac Lesions
- Ostial common iliac artery lesions will often require kissing balloon technique with a balloon placed in contralateral common iliac artery
- Carefully choose balloon size and position to not overdistend distal aorta

Proximal Common Iliac Lesions
- Non-ostial proximal common iliac lesions can often be angioplastied or stented without entering contralateral iliac artery

Distal Common Iliac and Proximal External Iliac
- Try not to stent across internal iliac artery (IIA) ostium unless necessary
- Abrupt occlusion of IIA ostium can lead to buttock claudication

Middle External Iliac Lesions
- External iliac lesions are prone to post angioplasty dissection
- If lesion looks like good candidate for Percutaneous Transluminal Angioplasty (PTA), may do PTA
- However, if has complex features, then probably best to primarily stent

Distal External Iliac Lesions
- Try not to stent across inguinal ligament
  - Increases risk of external compression of stent

Postangioplasty Arteriogram
- Check at least 2 views, such as AP and contralateral oblique

Postangioplasty Intravascular Pressures
- Place end -hole catheter across lesion into distal aorta
  - Obtain pressure measurement proximal (with catheter) and distal (with sheath) to lesion

Self-Expanding Stents
- In general, self-expanding stents have advantage of greater flexibility and ability to be placed from contralateral approach

Balloon Expandable Stents
- In general, balloon expandable stents tend to have less flexibility, but greater radial force and ability for very precise positioning
- For hand-crimped stents, use balloon made for stents or stent may slip off

Post-Procedure

Things to Do
- Bed rest x 6 to 8 hours and overnight observation in hospital
- Aspirin 325 mg p.o. each day
- Check femoral and foot pulses or Doppler signals
- Schedule follow-up appointment

Common Problems & Complications
- Puncture site complications
- Elastic recoil and acute or delayed thrombosis of angioplasty or stent site
- Excessive arterial dissection and arterial rupture
- Stent malposition, migration, dislodgement and infection

Selected References
1. Smith JC et al: Angioplasty or stent placement in the proximal common iliac artery: Is protection or the contralateral side necessary? JVIR 12:1395-8, 2001
2. Reyes R et al: Treatment of chronic iliac artery occlusions with guidewire recanalization and primary stent placement. JVIR 8:1049-55, 1997
3. Sapoval MR et al: Self-expandable stents for the treatment of iliac artery obstructive lesions: Long-term success and prognostic factors. AJR 166:1173-9, 1996

Leg Arterial Thrombolysis

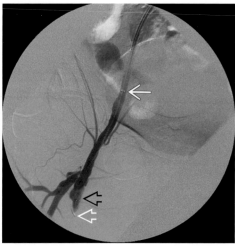

Thrombosed right lower leg graft: (White arrow), sheath placed from contralateral approach. (Black open arrow), indicates proximal graft. (White open arrow) indicates wire being placed into thrombus

Key Facts
- Procedure definition: Dissolution of clot in arteries or grafts
- Clinical setting triggering procedure: Lower extremity ischemia
- Best procedure approach: Depends on vessel, contralateral approach
- Most feared complications: Intracranial hemorrhage, GI bleeding, reperfusion syndrome
- Expected outcome: Restoration of flow through artery or graft

Pre-Procedure
Indications
- Acute or acute-on-chronic lower extremity ischemia, acute thrombosis of lower extremity arterial bypass graft, post angioplasty thrombosis
Contraindications
- Contraindication to thrombolytics
  - Irreversible ischemia, brain pathology (stroke, tumor) in past 2 months, active internal bleeding, major trauma, surgery, biopsy in past 2 weeks, coagulation defects, uncontrolled severe hypertension, embolus with cardiac source, pregnancy
Getting Started
- Things to Check
  - Status of leg, risk factors for thrombolysis
  - Baseline labs: CBC, creatinine, coagulation profile, baseline fibrinogen
  - History of peripheral vascular procedures, anatomy of bypass grafts
- Equipment List
  - One wall needle, standard wire, Terumo glidewire, heavy duty wire
  - Catheters
    - 5 Fr pigtail or Omni for preliminary aortogram and runoff exam
    - Selective catheter for selecting thrombosed vessel
    - Multi-side-hole thrombolysis catheter set includes catheter, occluding wire, and Tuohy-Borst hemostatic valve

Leg Arterial Thrombolysis

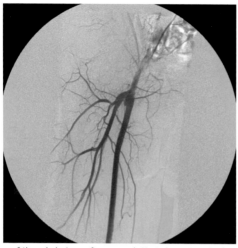

After 4 hours of thrombolysis, graft reopened. Next, inspect entire lower extremity vascular system to determine cause of thrombosis, and evaluate for possible emboli.

- Infusion wire or microinfusion catheter for coaxial administration
  o Sheath
    - If contralateral use Arrow Flex sheath, Balkan sheath
  o Medications
    - Conscious sedation, heparin, thrombolytic (alteplase - rtPA, Reteplase r-PA), aspirin, GPIIb/IIIa inhibitors (Integrilin, ReoPro)
  o Pump(s) for arterial infusion

Procedure
Patient Position/Location
- Supine, angiographic room
Procedure Steps
- Contralateral femoral artery, single wall puncture
- Aortogram and runoff examination
  o Get all relevant information of vasculature, information needed for surgical procedure if thrombolysis not successful
- Attempt to cross occlusion: Easy if fresh clot, more difficult in chronic clot, inability to cross predicts poor success
- Multi-side-hole catheter - length of side holes matched to occlusion length
- Pulse thrombolytic 0.2-0.4 cc Q 20 sec, TB syringe, forceful injection
  o tPA 2-5 mg in 20 cc of NS
  o Reteplase 3-5 units in 20 cc of NS
  o Heparin 2,500 unit IV bolus, begin on infusion of 500 units/hr
- After administration, evaluate angiographically, repeat if necessary
- Reevaluate, if continued thrombosis, move to infusion
- Infusion through pulse-spray catheter, but more advantageous to place end-hole catheter in proximal thrombus infuse thrombolytic, avoids stasis from catheter, particularly good if some flow reestablished
- Extensive clot, coaxial infusion with infusion wire or microcatheter

Leg Arterial Thrombolysis

- Catheter secured to the skin, dressing placed, infusion begun, if using coaxial system divide infusion
- Infusion rate
  - tPA: 0.5-1.0 mg/hr (10 mg/500 cc NS (0.02mg/ml), 25-50cc/hr)
  - Reteplase 0.25-1.0 U/hr (10U/1000 cc of NS (.01U/cc), 25-100cc/hr)
  - Heparin no more than 500 units/hr
- Reevaluate patient in 4-12 hours or when clinical situation demands
- Treat cause of thrombosis with endovascular methods or surgery

Alternative Procedures/Therapies
- Radiological
  - Thrombectomy devices, suction aspiration
- Surgical
  - Thrombectomy, bypass grafts

Post-Procedure
Things to Do
- Infusion therapy requires ICU
  - Frequent checks of VS, groin, distal pulses, perfusion, movement, sensation
  - Bleeding watch: Hematest stools, neurologic checks, minimize venous punctures
  - Labs q 4 hours: CBC, fibrinogen, PT, PTT, INR, PTT 1.25-1.5 control

Things to Avoid
- **NO** IM injections

Common Problems & Complications
Problems
- Clinical status of limb deteriorates
  - Usually represent emboli which will improve with further lysis
  - Reevaluate angiographically, may need surgery

Complications
- Severe
  - Intracranial hemorrhage, GI bleeding, compartment syndrome
- Other complications
  - Embolization into distal vessels – usually treated with more thrombolysis, bleeding at puncture site

Selected References
1. Shlansky-Goldberg R: Platelet aggregation inhibitors for use in peripheral vascular interventions. JVIR 13:229-46, 2002
2. Semba et al: Thrombolytic therapy with the use of Alteplase (rt-PA) in peripheral arterial occlusive disease. JVIR 11:149-61, 2000
3. Davidian MM et al: Initial results of Reteplase in the treatment of acute lower extremity arterial occlusions. JVIR 11:289-94, 2000

Lower Extremity Arteriogram

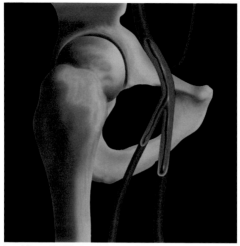

Right anterior oblique (RAO) view helps to demonstrate CFA bifurcation and DFA origin. This is important for treatment planning. DFA origin is common site of stenoses.

Key Facts
- Peripheral vascular disease (PVD) is most common indication
- Goal is to determine cause of symptoms as well as potential percutaneous and surgical treatment options
- Routine femoral arteriogram typically includes aorta from renal arteries downward and iliac arteries

Pre-Procedure
Indications
- PVD
- Knee dislocation
- Penetrating trauma

Contraindications
- Uncorrectable bleeding diathesis
- Bilateral common femoral artery (CFA) occlusions
  - Procedure can still be done from arm
- Moderate renal failure is relative contraindication
  - Hydrate
  - Consider other nephroprotective agents
  - Minimize contrast load
  - Sometimes can limit study to most symptomatic leg
  - Consider only leg arteriogram and skip aortogram if strong bilateral femoral pulses and triphasic waveforms

Getting Started
- Things to Check
  - If patient on heparin or Coumadin
  - Creatinine, platelets and INR
  - Which leg is more symptomatic
    - Puncture other side
  - Check femoral pulses

Lower Extremity Arteriogram

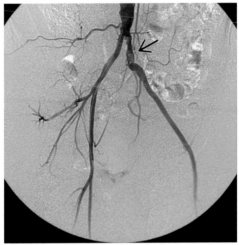

RAO view increases visualization of left CIA bifurcation and right CFA bifurcation. Note: Bulky atherosclerotic plaque in left CIA (arrow).

- Equipment List
  - 65 cm long, 5 French pigtail, tennis racquet or Omni Flush catheter
  - Hook-shaped tip catheter when will select contralateral iliac artery

Procedure

Patient Position/Location
- Supine

Equipment Preparation
- Flush catheters, wires and sheath

Procedure Steps
- Place a 5 French sheath in CFA
- Place a pigtail or similar multi-side-hole catheter in aorta just distal to expected location of renal arteries
- Obtain an abdominal aortogram
  - Usual injection rate is 15 cc per second for a total of 30 cc contrast (15/30)
  - A single AP view is usually adequate
  - Decreasing source to image distance (SID) will increase the field of view

Iliac Artery Arteriogram
- Pull catheter down to distal aorta and obtain bilateral oblique views of pelvis with at least 30 degrees of obliquity
  - Usual injection rate is 10 cc per second for a total of 20 cc (10/20)
  - RAO (Right Anterior Oblique) view shows left common iliac artery bifurcation
  - RAO also shows right CFA bifurcation
  - Oblique views in this region are important
  - Deep femoral artery (DFA) has a posterolateral origin from CFA
- Stenoses often occur at origin of DFA and superficial femoral artery (SFA)
- Complete the study with a simultaneous bilateral lower extremity

Lower Extremity Arteriogram

- Arteriogram with catheter in distal aorta
  - Or select contralateral external iliac and do a selective arteriogram of that leg
- If iliac arteries are patent and main site of disease is infrapopliteal, a selective arteriogram may be of benefit
- If percutaneous and surgical options can be determined with a nonselective study, then this is adequate
- By "selective" lower extremity arteriogram, it is meant that catheter tip is in ipsilateral external iliac artery of lower extremity that is imaged
- Selective study, images only one side at a time
- Ipsilateral leg is imaged by injection thru sidearm of sheath

Popliteal Bifurcation
- Open interosseus space between fibula and tibia by turning patient's leg or by obliquing C-arm
- Not uncommon that 2 pictures of differing obliquity are necessary to get adequate views this region

Infrapopliteal Arteries
- Important for treatment planning
- Cortex of tibia and fibula can obscure vessels
- Oblique imaging can open up interosseous space
- Transcatheter intraarterial nitroglycerin (IA NTG) 150 to 200 microgram boluses can be helpful to maximize vasodilation and opacification
  - NTG has a short half-life
  - Repeated boluses may be necessary

Foot Arteriogram
- Use digital subtraction angiography and collimate
- Visipaque contrast is well tolerated and usually does not cause pain
  - Thus patient is less likely to move
- Increase dose of iodinated contrast to increase vessel opacification
- Selective angiography improves visualization of foot arteries
- NTG 100 to 300 microgram boluses are helpful for vasodilation
- Avoid excess plantarflexion and tight taping over dorsalis pedis artery
- Warm foot at least by covering with blanket, because cold leads to vasoconstriction, pain, and movement

Post-Procedure
Things to Do
- Obtain hemostasis, bed rest for 6 hours, monitor puncture site and pulses

Common Problems & Complications
- Inadequate opacification of arteries in symptomatic region
- Puncture site complications such as dissection and hematoma
- Iliac or femoral artery thrombosis

Selected References
1. Gates J et al: Optimized diagnostic angiography in high-risk patients with severe peripheral vascular disease. Radiographics 20:121-33, 2000
2. Hartnell G et al: MR angiography compared with digital subtraction angiography. AJR 175:1188-9, 2000
3. Alson MD et al: Pedal arterial imaging. JVIR 8:9-18, 1997

Mesenteric Angiography

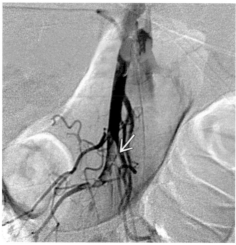

Close-up of SMA embolus (arrow).

Key Facts
- Mesenteric ischemia, gastrointestinal bleeding and as part of a hepatic chemoembolization procedure are most common indications
  - This chapter focuses on mesenteric ischemia
- Routine mesenteric arteriogram typically includes abdominal aortogram PA and lateral, as well as selective catheterization of superior mesenteric artery (SMA) and sometimes inferior mesenteric artery (IMA)

Pre-Procedure
<u>Indications</u>
- Acute and chronic mesenteric ischemia (AMI and CMI)
- Gastrointestinal bleeding
- As part of hepatic chemoembolization
- Arterial portography

<u>Contraindications</u>
- Uncorrectable bleeding diathesis

<u>Getting Started</u>
- Things to Check
  - Check PT, PTT, platelets, hemoglobin, creatinine, lactic acid
  - Check femoral pulses
  - There are multiple causes of mesenteric ischemia
    - Mesenteric artery embolus (MAE) is usually seen in association with myocardial infarction and/or atrial fibrillation
    - MAE is most common cause of AMI
    - MAE typically occurs in SMA
    - Mesenteric artery thrombosis (MAT) typically occurs at SMA origin and is associated with underlying atherosclerosis
    - Cholesterol crystal embolization (CCE) may occur following angiography procedures such as coronary or renal artery angioplasty
    - Abdominal aorta dissection may extend into SMA and IMA and cause mesenteric ischemia

Mesenteric Angiography

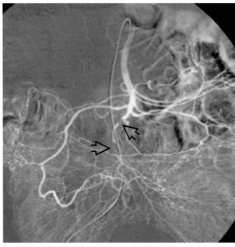

Two emboli are seen as filling defects (open arrows) in the superior mesenteric artery.
The patient had severe abdominal pain, atrial fibrillation and a low INR.

- Non-occlusive mesenteric ischemia (NOMI) is associated with systemic hypotension, mesenteric vasospasm and vasopressor medications
- Mesenteric venous thrombosis (MVT) may occur due to a hypercoagulable state, cirrhosis with portal hypertension, pancreatitis or following surgery such as splenectomy
- Angiography findings may include delayed or non-visualization of mesenteric veins and thrombus in veins
  - AMI typically occurs in elderly patients and is associated with complaints of pain out of proportion to tenderness elicited by palpation, diarrhea, elevated white blood cell count, elevated lactic acid
  - Additional findings may include sudden onset of abdominal pain, abdominal distention due to ileus, hemoccult positive stools, respiratory failure, elevated amylase, and emboli to other locations e.g. extremities
  - CT findings of AMI include SMA stenosis or occlusion, bowel wall thickening and nonenhancement, pneumatosis intestinalis and portal vein air or mesenteric vein thrombosis
  - CMI is associated with elderly patients that have extensive atherosclerosis in other areas such as coronaries, carotids or lower extremities, postprandial pain, fear of eating and weight loss
  - Ultrasound may show proximal mesenteric arteries, but is limited due to bowel gas in critically ill patients
  - CT and CT angiography can demonstrate proximal portions of mesenteric arteries and veins, but has limited visualization of more distal vessels
    - Catheter angiography remains the gold standard for evaluation of the mesenteric vasculature
- Equipment List

Mesenteric Angiography

- 5 French sheath and 65 cm long, pigtail, racquet or Omni Flush catheter
- Catheter with a reversed curve upon itself such as a Simmons #2 or #3 and Sos Omni Selective

Procedure
Patient Position
- Supine

Procedure Steps
- Place a pigtail or similar catheter in aorta just above celiac artery
- Obtain abdominal aortogram in PA and lateral view
  - 20 cc per second for a total of 40 cc is a routine injection rate
  - Best view for proximal celiac artery and SMA is lateral projection
- IMA arises from anterior aspect of distal abdominal aorta and is often not well visualized on aortograms when pigtail catheter is near SMA
  - Contrast is heavier than blood and layers within posterior aortic lumen, as can be seen on lateral aortogram
- Place pigtail catheter at level of ostium of IMA and obtain "flush" arteriogram of IMA with PA and steep RAO views
  - May provide adequate visualization of IMA and preclude need for selective catheterization
- If IMA not adequately imaged with earlier flush arteriogram, then can be selectively catheterized
  - May be beneficial to obtain images of IMA early in procedure as contrast in urinary bladder may obscure IMA territory in patients that do not have a Foley catheter
- If proximal SMA is patent, then selectively catheterize SMA with a reversed curved tip catheter
- Do a hand injection to check position, assess flow and plan injection rate
- Obtain arteriograms in PA and oblique projections, making sure to obtain images of entire SMA territory
  - 6 cc per second for 30 cc total is a routine injection rate in SMA

Post-Procedure
- Obtain hemostasis, bed rest for 6 hours, monitor puncture site and pulses

Common Problems & Complications
- Suboptimal opacification of arteries due to patient motion or difficulties with selective catheterization
- Puncture site complications and iatrogenic injury of mesenteric arteries

Selected References
1. Cognet F et al: Chronic mesenteric ischemia: imaging and percutaneous treatment. Radiographics 22: 863-79, 2002
2. Song S-Y et al: Collateral pathways in celiac axis stenosis: Angiographic-Spiral CT correlation. Radiographics 22:881-93, 2002
3. Horton KM et al: Multi-detector row CT of mesenteric ischemia: Can it be done? Radiographics 21:1463-73, 2001

Perclose

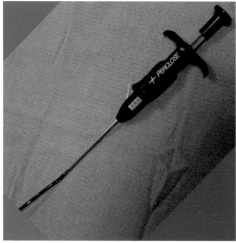

The Perclose device is used to percutaneously suture common femoral arteriotomies to obtain hemostasis.

Key Facts
- Perclose device is used following angiography to suture common femoral arteriotomy site
- Perclose is effective at obtaining hemostasis
- Suture is deployed thru same puncture site as used for angiography
- Facilitates early anticoagulation following thrombolysis or stenting
- Also facilitates early ambulation and ability of patient to go home
- Meticulous sterile technique is important

Pre-Procedure

Indications
- To obtain hemostasis after common femoral artery (CFA) puncture

Contraindications
- Skin infection overlying puncture site
- Femoral artery stenosis greater than 50%
- Heavily calcified CFA such that calcium is fluoroscopically visible
- Femoral arteries less than 5 mm in diameter
- Pregnancy
- Superficial or deep femoral artery puncture
- In extremely large patients, the puncture site may be too deep to be reached by Perclose device

Getting Started
- Things to Check
  - Check that puncture area does not appear infected
- Equipment List
  - 0.035", angled tip, 150 cm long glidewire
  - Perclose device comes with knot tier and knot clincher

Procedure

Patient Position
- Supine

Perclose

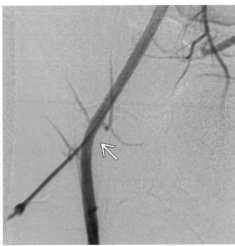

Contrast is injected thru sidearm of common femoral artery (CFA) sheath to check location of arterial entry (arrow) relative to CFA bifurcation and side branches.

Equipment Preparation
- Flush the Perclose device and wipe the glidewire

Procedure Steps
- Place the fluoroscope into a 45 degree ipsilateral oblique view
  - Allows visualization of sheath entry into CFA and of CFA branches
- Watch under fluoro as contrast is injected thru sheath
  - Obtain a last image hold or an arteriogram of CFA region
- Ideally, CFA entry site should be at least 5 mm proximal to CFA bifurcation and away from any large side branches

Glidewire and Device Placement
- Glidewire is placed thru sheath to level of diaphragm
- Sheath is removed and guidewire must be kept wet
- Perclose device is passed over guidewire
- Perclose device is advanced up until site of guidewire exit from perclose device is at skin level
- Guidewire is removed
- Advance perclose device at a similar angle as angiogram needle was originally inserted

Opening Footplates
- Device is inserted into artery until flow is seen to come out of side spout known as marker lumen
- Open footplates by pulling lever upward
- Device is gently withdrawn until footplates are snug against inner surface of anterior wall of artery
- Device should be held at a 45 degree angle

Deploying Needles
- Needles can now be deployed by pushing plunger downwards
- Pressure should be maintained on plunger for 10 seconds

Cutting Suture Away from Needles
- Plunger is withdrawn and suture threads are held gently taut
- Plunger can be turned sideways to make threads more visible

- Suture threads are then cut adjacent to needles

Using Knot Tier
- Perclose device is withdrawn until suture threads are visible
- Manufacturer recommends that sutures be wetted
- Caudal thread is called #1, and is pulled thru loop #1 on knot clincher
- It is important from here until end of procedure not to touch suture #1
  - Because tension on suture #1 at this point will prematurely lock knot
- Suture #2 is then pulled thru loop #2 of knot clincher and then pulled thru metal trapezoidal loop of knot pusher
  - Suture #2 is then wrapped around index finger of physician's left hand
  - Tension applied to suture #2 should be along same axis as original CFA needle puncture
- Perclose device is now removed from artery
- Distal part of suture #2 thread is wrapped around left hand index finger
- Simultaneously as device is being removed, increased tension is applied to suture #2
- Knot pusher is now pushed so that it slides down suture #2 until contacting anterior wall of artery
  - Gentle pressure is applied with knot pusher
- Knot pusher is removed to check for hemostasis
  - Usually hemostasis will be obtained by this time
- Now, lock knot by pulling on suture #1
- Usually a slight "jump" is felt when it locks
- Suture is then cut with scissors at skin level
  - Skin at puncture site is pushed downward with hemostat encircling sutures #1 and #2 as the threads are pulled upwards
  - Cut as close to skin entry level as possible
- Goal is to cut suture threads as short as possible so that they will retract further below skin level

Post-Procedure
Things to Do
- Can usually ambulate in 2½ hours and discharge home in 3 hours
- No shower for at least 24 hours and site should not be submerged for at least 5 days

Common Problems & Complications
Complications
- Bleeding
- Lack of needle capture
- Infection
- Iatrogenic arterial stenosis
- Failure to obtain hemostasis
- Pain at puncture site

Selected References
1. Morris PP et al: Neurointerventional experience with an arteriotomy suture device. AJNR 20:1706-9, 1999
2. Duda SH et al: Suture-mediated closure of antegrade femoral arterial access sites in patients with full anticoagulation therapy. RJ 210:47-52, 1999

Puncture Site Compression

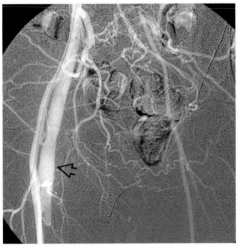

Right femoral Arteriovenous Fistula (AVF) following cardiac catheterization with right femoral puncture. Note: Venous filling of right common femoral vein (open arrow) during arterial phase.

Key Facts
- Minimum compression time femoral or brachial is 12 minutes
- With hematoma risk factors, correct problem and/or compress longer
- Brachial artery is more difficult to compress than femoral

Pre-Procedure
<u>Indications</u>
- Hemostasis must be obtained at all arterial puncture sites

<u>Contraindications</u>
- Markedly elevated ACT following heparin
- Sheath needs to be used for other procedure immediately to follow

<u>Getting Started</u>
- Equipment List
  - Sterile gloves, 4 x 4 gauze and absorbent towels

<u>Risk Factors for Hematoma</u>
- Anticoagulation with heparin or Coumadin
- Severe hypertension
  - Can treat with Versed, labetalol or hydralazine
- Chronic oral steroids
  - Compress longer than usual, e.g., 15 to 20 minutes
- Brachial and axillary arterial puncture
  - Pulse in upper arm is more mobile than femoral pulse
- High puncture site
  - E.g. external iliac artery puncture
  - Risk for massive occult bleeding into pelvis
  - Compress longer than usual, e.g. 20 minutes
  - Fluoro over contrast-filled bladder to check for displacement by hematoma
- Low puncture site
  - Typically a superficial femoral artery puncture

Puncture Site Compression

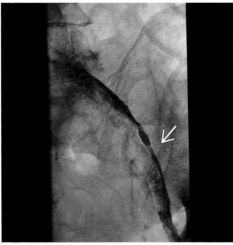

Left iliac artery dissection. No spontaneous flow from sheath placed into dissection. Sheath (white arrow) was withdrawn and dissection spontaneously resolved. Contralateral approach can be used to place pigtail catheter in aorta for pelvis arteriogram.

- o Increased risk for hematoma, pseudoaneurysm and arteriovenous fistula formation
- o More difficult at this site to obtain good compression because there is no bone below artery
- Large sheath
- Calcified femoral artery
  - o Less elastic recoil than normal femoral arteries
  - o Key to success is prolonged compression
- Abnormal coagulation status
  - o E.g. with liver (elevated INR) and renal disease (decreased platelet function)
  - o Can give Vit. K, FFP or platelets, to decrease risk of bleeding
- Obesity

Procedure
Patient Position
- Supine

Procedure Steps
- Try to feel pulse when compressing
- Usually will be able to feel pulse when compressing

Hand Placement
- Goal is to compress actual site where needle entered
  - o Helpful to also compress just proximal to where needle entered
- Compression is typically done with ring, middle and index fingers
  - o Compress with fingertips, not with gauze

Usual Sequence of Steps
- Take your lead off
- Put on sterile gown (optional) and sterile gloves
- Feel location of pulse before removing sheath

Puncture Site Compression

- Look at clock and figure out when 15 minutes will have elapsed
  - This is your target time
  - Make sure that that clock is clearly visible
- Compress firmly for first 5 minutes
  - Goal is to obtain hemostasis, but not to occlude flow
- Ask patient how he/she is doing and if leg feels normal
  - If complains of pain in foot, check pulse or Doppler signal of foot
  - It is possible that artery is being over compressed
  - Try to compress gently but still maintain hemostasis
- Compress for a total of around 15 minutes
- As you get ready to stop compressing, give patient instructions
  - Tell him/her not to lift head and not talk for 5 minutes
  - Remind him/her of importance of bed rest
- Remove pressure of compression very gradually
  - Do not withdraw hand abruptly

Post-Procedure
Things to Do
- Be gentle when cleaning off Betadine, cleaning site can cause rebleeding
- Bed rest x 6 hours without moving leg
- Check BP, pulse, bilateral foot pulse or Doppler, groin bleed/hematoma q 15 minutes x 2, q 30 minutes x 2, q 1 hour x 5
- Notify doctor if any changes
- Apply pressure x 15 minutes if bleeding or hematoma occurs

Common Problems & Complications
Management of Groin Hematoma
- Compress firmly over expected site of pulse
- Goal is to compress hematoma so that it softens and pulse becomes palpable
- Once pulse is palpated, compress for an additional 15 minutes
  - Ultrasound can be used to locate pulse
- Outline hematoma with a marker and instruct nurse to compress site and to have you notified if hematoma gets any larger
  - CT scan of pelvis can be obtained
- Send for a type and screen as well as for hemoglobin level
- If hemostasis cannot be obtained, surgery should be consulted
- Hematomas with brachial puncture can compress median nerve
- Hematomas with axillary puncture can compress brachial plexus
  - Neurovascular status of hand should be evaluated and followed
  - Vascular surgery should be consulted with upper arm hematomas
- Prolonged bleeding
- Hematoma
- Painful hematoma e.g. of rectus sheath
- Pseudoaneurysm
- Thrombosis of external iliac, femoral artery or brachial artery

Selected References
1. Reeder SB et al: Low-dose thrombin injection to treat iatrogenic femoral artery pseudoaneurysms. AJR 177:595-8, 2001
2. McNeil NL et al: Sonographically Guided Percutaneous Thrombin Injection Versus Sonographically Guided Compression for Femoral Artery Pseudoaneurysms. AJR 176: 459-62, 2001
3. Trerotola SO et al: CT and anatomic study of postcatheterization hematomas. Radiographics 11: 247-58, 1991

Renal Artery Stent

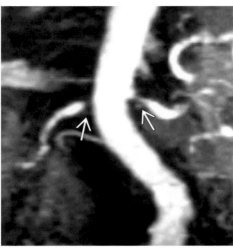

Magnetic resonance arteriogram (MRA) maximum intensity projection (MIP) in coronal plane shows severe bilateral proximal renal artery stenosis (white arrows).

Key Facts
- Percutaneous transluminal renal artery angioplasty and stenting (PTRAS) is most commonly done for treatment of refractory hypertension and renal insufficiency due to renal artery stenosis (RAS)
- PTRAS can be done with 0.035" and smaller guidewire systems such as 0.014"
  - This chapter will focus on use of a 0.035" guidewire system

Pre-Procedure
Indications
- Refractory hypertension (HTN) due to ostial renal artery stenosis (RAS)
- Renal failure due to RAS
- Salvage of a poor renal artery angioplasty result

Contraindications
- Uncorrectable bleeding diathesis
- Long segment renal artery occlusion
- Diffuse small branch stenoses
- Renal artery (Ra) 4 mm or less in diameter
- Small atrophic kidney

Getting Started
- Things to Check
  - Clinical history and list of blood pressure medications
  - Bleeding history, platelets, PT, PTT, INR
  - Confirm vascular surgery backup and/or covered stents available
  - Administer cefazolin 1 gram IV
  - Renal MRA is very helpful for demonstration of RAS location and approximate severity
    - Axial images are helpful to show orientation of Ra relative to aorta and thus for planning optimal obliquity with fluoroscopy
- Equipment List
  - Short 8 French sheath or long 6 French sheath

Renal Artery Stent

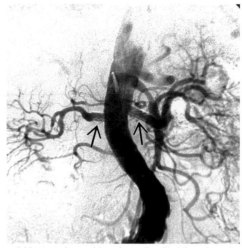

Balloon expandable stents (arrows) have been placed in bilateral renal arteries which are now widely patent.

- o Sos-omni selective 5 French catheter
- o Wholey guidewire for crossing Ra stenosis
- o 0.035" Rosen (1.5 mm J-tip) 200 cm long guidewire
- o 4 mm or 5mm diameter balloon, 2 cm long for predilation
- o 5 to 7 mm diameter balloon with premounted balloon expandable stent
- o 8 French guiding catheter with multipurpose tip and rotating hemostatic valve for contrast injection around guidewire and balloon

Procedure
Patient Position
- Supine
Procedure Steps
- Place 8 French sheath in right common femoral artery
- Administer 3,000 units of heparin intravenously
- Obtain a diagnostic aortagram with pigtail or tennis racquet catheter in AP and 5 degrees LAO for left Ra and 30 degrees LAO for right Ra
  - o Choice of obliquity can also be guided by orientation of Raa as seen on axial MRI images
  - o Try to determine optimal view for visualization of Ra origins
- Select main Ra e.g. with Sos-omni selective catheter
- Inject 100-200 micrograms nitroglycerin thru catheter, into Ra
- Place Wholey guidewire into distal Ra and advance catheter across lesion
  - o Be gentle, as Raa are very prone to spasm and perforation
- Exchange for a 0.035" Rosen (1.5 mm J-tip) 200 cm long guidewire
- Keep guidewire position fixed for remainder of procedure to avoid spasm
- Estimate size of renal artery, length of stenosis, location of adjacent branch vessels and for presence of Ra ostial plaque extension into aorta
- Predilate main renal artery with a 4 or 5 mm balloon, usually 2 cm long
- Select appropriate diameter and length balloon expandable stent
- Advance stent thru rotating valve and multipurpose guiding catheter

Renal Artery Stent

- Stagger tip of balloon, stent and guiding catheter for a more streamlined entry into main renal artery
- Advance premounted stent close to renal artery origin
- Perform hand injections of contrast thru guiding catheter to further define orientation of Ra origin and to optimize stent positioning
- Advance balloon with premounted stent into Ra and across stenosis
- Confirm optimal orientation of balloon
  o Will be view in which balloon appears longest
  o Helps to make sure stent will be correctly positioned
- Confirm stent correctly positioned relative to renal artery stenosis and to renal artery ostium/aorta
  o Stent will often project 1 or 2 mm into aorta to cover ostial plaque
  o Try to avoid placing proximal end of stent further into aorta
- Inflate balloon to deploy stent
- Obtain Ra arteriogram by injection through guiding catheter
- Check appearance of Ra stent and redilate if necessary

Post-Procedure
Things to Do
- Bed rest for 6 hours with overnight observation in ICU with monitoring of blood pressure, urine output and follow-up creatinine level
- Continue IV fluids which can be increased if the blood pressure decreases
- Aspirin 325 mg p.o. q day
- Prophylactic antibiotics may be given if patients undergo procedures that may cause bacteremia within next 4 weeks

Common Problems & Complications
- Unable to traverse RAS with guidewire
- Renal artery spasm
- Renal artery embolization with infarction of renal parenchyma
- Guidewire perforation of renal artery e.g. with subcapsular, perirenal or pararenal hematoma
- Rupture of renal artery by balloon or stent
- Misplacement of stent and dislodgement of stent e.g. stent slips off balloon
- Stent restenosis, thrombosis and infection
- Renal artery pseudoaneurysm
- Aortic dissection
- Cholesterol embolization with renal and/or intestinal infarction
- Acute renal failure

Selected References
1. Morris CS et al: Nonsurgical treatment of acute iatrogenic renal artery injuries occurring after renal artery angioplasty and stenting. AJR 177: 1353-7, 2001
2. Bukhari RH et al: Bilateral renal artery stent infection and pseudoaneurysm formation. JVIR 11:337-41, 2000
3. Kim PA et al: Fluoroscopic landmarks for optimal visualization of proximal renal arteries. JVIR 10:37-9, 1999

Renal Artery Embolization

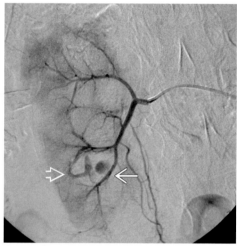

*Renal arteriogram demonstrates **arteriovenous fistula** (open arrow) and **pseudoaneurysm** (arrow) causing massive hematuria following percutaneous stone removal.*

Key Facts
- Most common indication for renal artery embolization (RAE) is hemorrhage due to percutaneous renal procedures such as biopsy, nephrostomy and nephrolithotomy
  - Chapter will focus on this indication
  - Goal is to stop bleeding while minimizing infarction of normal kidney
- 5 French end-hole catheters and stainless steel coils are used for embolization of large vessels
- Microcatheters and microcoils are helpful for small distal branches

Pre-Procedure
Indications
- Iatrogenic massive hemorrhage following percutaneous renal procedures
- Trauma related hemorrhage
- Preoperative devascularization of renal cell carcinoma
- Hemorrhagic angiomyolipoma of kidney
- Severe refractory nephrotic syndrome

Contraindications
- Uncorrectable bleeding diathesis

Getting Started
- Things to Check
  - Bleeding history, platelets, PT, PTT, INR and creatinine
  - Administer prophylactic antibiotics
  - Review CT scan as may indicate likely site of hemorrhage
    - If abnormalities not seen on routine angiographic views, selective views at site of probable bleeding on CT or ultrasound can be helpful
- Equipment List
  - 5 French (Fr) sheath and 65 cm pigtail or tennis racquet catheter
  - Cobra or Simmons 5 French catheter

Renal Artery Embolization

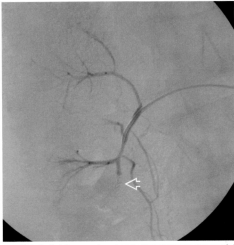

Arteriovenous fistula *(white arrow) and* ***pseudoaneurysm*** *successfully embolized with coils. There was no further bleeding.*

- Only endhole catheters are used for embolization
- Catheters with sideholes are not used because embolic material may exit thru sideholes and infarct nontarget tissue
  - 0.035" angled tip glidewire to select target artery
  - 0.035" Bentson guidewire to use as a "pusher" for coils
  - Stainless steel coils for deployment thru 0.035" or 0.038" lumen catheters
    - These coils are larger and tend to achieve target vessel thrombosis more rapidly than with microcoils
    - However, 5 Fr catheters more likely to cause spasm in small vessels
  - Microcatheters and microcoils may be used if selective catheterization of distal vessels is necessary
    - Requires use of rotating hemostatic valve and pressurized saline flush bag attached to hub of 5 Fr catheter and microcatheter

Procedure
Patient Position
- Supine
Procedure Steps
- Place 5 French sheath into femoral artery
- Obtain aortagram and check size and number of renal arteries (Ra), and for abnormalities such as pseudoaneurysm, arteriovenous fistula (AVF) and extravasation
- Catheterize Ra with 5 Fr endhole catheter and obtain renal arteriogram
- If technically feasible, perform embolization with this catheter
- If necessary, use microcatheter to reach more distal sites
- Be gentle with guidewires as renal artery is prone to spasm
- Select appropriate diameter and length coil
  - Desirable coil size is 1 mm larger than vessel in which deployed
  - Too small of a coil may migrate distally

Renal Artery Embolization

- o Too long of a coil may protrude proximally and reflux into aorta
- Insert coil into catheter and then advance coil thru catheter by pushing with back end of a Bentson guidewire for the 1st 30 cm of catheter length
- Then turn Bentson wire around and use soft/front end to "push" coil
- Deploy coils with a gentle "tap-tap-tap" motion on Bentson guidewire
    - o This stabilizes catheter and facilitates tight curling of coil as deployed
    - o If just push coil straight out, more likely to cause catheter to back out of vessel and coil less likely to form/curl well
- Can use guidewire to gently pack coils together to promote thrombosis
- Can supplement with gelfoam embolization
- Inject contrast to check thrombotic effect of coils
- Deploy additional coils or gelfoam if necessary

Embolization of Renal Cell Carcinoma
- Should be done within 24 hours of scheduled surgery
- If use coils in distal main renal artery, make sure leave enough room for surgeon to clamp main renal artery

Post-Procedure
- Bed rest for 6 hours
- Follow symptoms, urine output, blood pressure, pulse and hemoglobin level to check for recurrent bleeding
- Treat symptoms of post embolization syndrome e.g. with antiemetics for nausea, tylenol for fever, opioids for pain and IV fluids

Common Problems & Complications
- Renal artery spasm
- Guidewire perforation of renal artery
- Nontarget renal embolization with infarction of renal parenchyma
- Nontarget embolization of adrenal gland, e.g. due to ethanol reflux
- Nontarget embolization with intestinal infarction
    - o Ethanol may reflux into aorta and pass into inferior mesenteric artery
- Coil migration with reflux of coil into aorta
- Coil migration with passage thru AVF and embolization to lung
- Acute renal failure
- Hypertension
- Postembolization syndrome with nausea, vomiting, fever, pain and leukocytosis
    - o More likely with RAE of large tumor than of focal bleeding site
- Renal abscess developing within infarcted tissue

Selected References
1. Dinkel HP et al: Blunt renal trauma: Minimally invasive management with microcatheter embolization experience in nine patients. Radiology 223:723-30, 2002
2. Centenera LV et al: Wide-necked saccular renal artery aneursym: Endovascular embolization with the Guglielmi detachable coil and temporary balloon occlusion of the aneursym neck. JVIR 9:513-6, 1998
3. Bakal CW et al: Value of preoperative renal artery embolization in reducing blood transfusion requirements during nephrectomy for renal cell carcinoma. JVIR 4:727-31, 1993

Thoracic Aorta Angiography

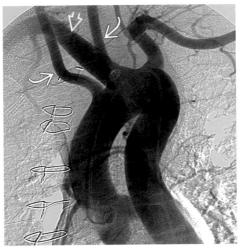

Thoracic aortography with an aberrant right subclavian artery (open arrow). Bilateral common carotid arteries (curved arrows).

Key Facts
- Most common indication for thoracic aorta angiography (TAA) is as part of a cerebral angiography diagnostic or therapeutic procedure
- Higher contrast rates and volumes and increased number of angiographic views are required for trauma evaluation
  - As CT has progressively taken on a larger role in evaluation of aortic trauma, the number of requests for TAA has decreased

Pre-Procedure
Indication
- Most common indication for TAA is as part of a cerebral angiography diagnostic or therapeutic procedure
  - Helps diagnose stenoses of great vessel origins and shows vertebral artery origins and sizes which facilitates choosing which one to catheterize
  - Obtaining both LAO (left anterior oblique) and RAO (right anterior oblique) views facilitates planning for endovascular procedures
  - When there is diffuse severe atherosclerotic disease with stenoses of great vessel origins, a carotid arteriogram can be performed with catheter in ascending thoracic aorta
- As part of evaluation of subclavian steal syndrome, thoracic outlet syndrome, vasculitis and other similar diseases
- Trauma with potential for injury of thoracic aorta or great vessels
  - CT is now often done as primary study for trauma
- Thoracic aorta stent graft placement
Contraindications
- Uncorrectable bleeding diathesis
Getting Started
- Things to Check
  - History of surgery or trauma to thoracic aorta
  - Check previous CT, if any, in trauma patients

Thoracic Aorta Angiography

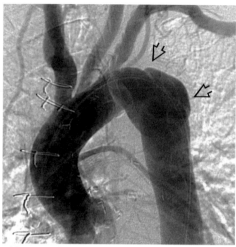

Left anterior oblique view shows transection of thoracic aorta (open arrows) following MVA. By visually following the contour of the aortic wall, the finding appears more obvious.

- o Check INR, PTT, platelets and creatinine
- Equipment List
  - o 5 French, 100 cm long, pigtail catheter is used for non-trauma TAA
  - o For evaluation of trauma, a 7 French catheter may be used to facilitate high contrast injection rates
  - o 3 mm J-tip, 145 cm long guidewire
  - o Use dense, nonionic, iodinated contrast e.g. Omnipaque (iohexol)

Procedure
Patient Position
- Supine

Procedure Steps
- Place sheath in right femoral artery
- Observe catheter with fluoroscopy as advance
- Place pigtail catheter in ascending thoracic aorta approximately midway between aortic valve and innominate artery
- Pigtail catheters have multiple sideholes which allow blood to enter distal catheter
  - o Always double flush when working above diaphragm
  - o Aspirate catheter forcefully before flushing with heparinized saline
  - o Work quickly
  - o Do not allow catheter to sit idle for prolonged amounts of time, as this may permit clots to form
- Perform a hand injection of contrast to check position of catheter relative to aortic valve and innominate artery as well as to evaluate rapidity of flow

Views
- LAO
  - o In general, this is best view to "open up the arch"
  - o If only get one view with a cerebral arteriogram, then get this view

- o 45 degrees LAO is a routine amount of obliquity
- o Obtaining an additional steeper LAO view, e.g. 60 degrees LAO, can be helpful for evaluation of trauma
- RAO view requires a large amount of obliquity to open up arch in this direction e.g. 75 degrees RAO
- PA
- For trauma, obtain at least 3 views with injection rates of 30 cc per second for a total of 60 cc with DSA (digital subtraction angiography)
- For nontrauma DSA evaluation, injection of 25 cc per second for a total of 40 cc is usually adequate

TAA Interpretation with Trauma
- Check aorta and great vessels for traumatic injuries such as pseudoaneurysm formation with discontinuity or irregularity of aortic contour
  - o Most often occurs immediately distal to left subclavian artery origin
  - o Injuries can be multiple
- Make sure descending aorta is visualized to level of diaphragm on at least one view
- Normal variants include ductus diverticulum and infundibulum ectasia of innominate and intercostal artery origins

TAA Interpretation for Non-Trauma Diseases
- Check for stenoses of great vessel origins
- Check anatomical site of origin of great vessels e.g. check if left carotid and left subclavian arteries arise directly from arch or from other vessels
- If flow is slow in a particular vessel, suspect a distal, severe stenosis or occlusion

Post-Procedure
Things to Do
- Bed rest x 6 hours

Common Problems & Complications
- An ectatic origin of brachiocephalic artery may lead to pigtail catheter passing into brachiocephalic artery
  - o Can get past this by advancing pigtail catheter over a guidewire or using a hockey-stick type tip catheter
- Puncture site complications
- Ischemic stroke
- Aortic rupture e.g. in patients with post-traumatic injury and in patients with Ehlers-Danlos syndrome

Selected References
1. Ho VB et al: Thoracic MR aortography: Imaging techniques and strategies. Radiographics 18:287-309, 1998
2. Fisher RG et al: Subtle or atypical injuries of thoracic aorta and brachiocephalic vessels in blunt thoracic trauma. Radiographics 17:835-49, 1997
3. Fisher RG et al: "Lumps" and "bumps" that mimic acute aortic and brachiocephalic vessel injury. Radiographics 17: 825-34, 1997

Trauma Embolization

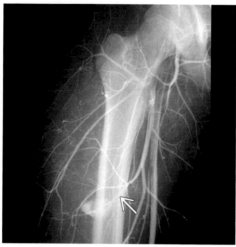

Stab wound to the thigh with large hematoma. Diagnostic angiogram performed from contralateral groin shows extravasation from profunda branch (arrow). Profunda branches can be safely embolized. More selective positioning will be performed prior to embolization.

Key Facts
- Procedure definition: Treatment of traumatic vascular injuries with embolization
- Clinical setting triggering procedure: Trauma patient with uncontrolled bleeding, CT scan demonstrating contrast extravasation
- Best procedure approach: Femoral artery
- Most feared complications: Embolization of non-target vessels, ischemia/ necrosis in area embolized
- Expected outcome: Control of bleeding with embolization

Pre-Procedure
Indications
- Patient with trauma (including iatrogenic) and uncontrolled bleeding
- CT scan demonstrating contrast extravasation
- Unstable patients without abdominal injury
Contraindications
- Unstable patients with abdominal trauma and positive lavage/US
Getting Started
- Things to Check
  - o Imaging studies, particularly CT for bleeding site
  - o Make sure patient is resuscitated or being resuscitated
  - o Large bore IVs, blood products, ICU type monitoring, crash cart
- Equipment List
  - o Standard wires, Terumo glidewire, sheath (use for catheterization and also for another source of access for fluid resuscitation if necessary)
  - o Catheters – depends on area to be studied
    - ▪ Pigtail, Omni catheter for nonselective overall evaluation
    - ▪ Selective catheters – Cobra, long reversed curve, headhunter
    - ▪ Microcatheters, microwires
  - o Embolization materials

Trauma Embolization

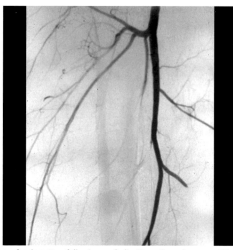

Injection in profunda artery following embolization. Branch responsible for bleeding has been embolized and there is no evidence of other branches supplying this area. Gelfoam was used for the embolization.

- Gelfoam often preferable in trauma; slurry or pledglets
- Coils/microcoils for very selective, focal embolization
- Particles, liquid embolics uncommonly used, more likely to cause ischemia

Procedure
Patient Position/Location
- Supine, angiographic equipment

Equipment Preparation
- Gelfoam cut into tiny pledglets for injection through catheter

Procedure Steps
- Perform global diagnostic angiogram of the target territory
- Look for evidence of vascular trauma
  - Extravasation, pseudoaneurysm, AVF, occlusion
- Selective angiography of traumatized arteries
  - Even if no bleeding seen on diagnostic angiogram usually a selective angiogram should be performed
- Extravasation /pseudoaneurysm, determine if embolization necessary
  - What will be consequences of occlusion? Vessel must be expendable
  - Is this vascular injury responsible for patient's condition?
  - Is there more than one bleeding site?
  - Is surgery or embolization more appropriate?
- Attempt to get catheter or microcatheter close to bleeding site, embolize as selectively as possible
  - Large vessel is bleeding, coils or a combination of coils and Gelfoam (a "Gelfoam sandwich") is preferable
  - Small artery, few particles of Gelfoam or a microcoil appropriate
  - In some cases, splenic injury, crush injury of pelvis; a less focused embolization with Gelfoam slurry maybe appropriate

Trauma Embolization

- o Splenic embolization maybe performed with proximal splenic artery embolization allowing collateral flow via short gastric arteries
- If collaterals can reconstitute the bleeding site, need to "close the back door", place catheter beyond the bleeding site, embolize across lesion
- Post embolization angiogram to make sure all bleeding controlled
- If bleeding from area with potential collaterals (pelvis) perform angiogram from other vessel to verify no contribution from other vessel

Alternative Procedures/Therapies
- Surgical
  - o Operation for control of bleeding, in many cases much less desirable
  - o Angiographic control of bleeding tends to be faster and more tissue sparing

Post-Procedure
Things to Do
- Aggressively treat hypothermia and coagulopathy
- If patient continues to bleed, reevaluate as necessary

Common Problems & Complications
Problems
- Difficulty in getting subselective for embolization
  - o Don't get to a "tour de force" subselective embolization and end up with a dead patient
  - o Embolize more proximally if necessary

Complications
- Severe
  - o Technical failure of procedure
  - o Embolization of vessels other than bleeding vessel
  - o Ischemia, necrosis in non-target tissues
  - o Abscess formation from ischemic/infarcted tissues
- Other complications
  - o Post embolization syndrome, particularly with solid organ embolization (liver, spleen)

Selected References
1. Dondelinger RF et al: Traumatic injuries: Radiological hemostatic intervention at admission. Eur Radiol 12:979-93, 2002
2. Maull KI: Current status of nonoperative management of liver injuries. World J Surg 25:1403-4, 2001
3. Sclafani SJA et al: Nonoperative salvage of computed tomography-diagnosed splenic injuries: Utilization of angiography for triage and embolization for hemostasis. J Trauma 39:818-27, 1995

Uterine Artery Embolization

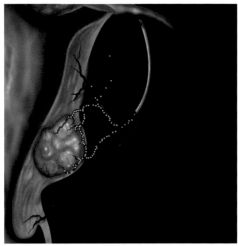

Selective catheterization right uterine artery. Hypervascular mass represents the fibroid. Catheterization performed with long reverse curve catheter.

Key Facts
- Procedure synonyms: UAE, UFE-uterine fibroid embolization
- Procedure definition: Embolization of uterine arteries
- Clinical setting triggering procedure: Severe menstrual bleeding, bulk symptoms-frequency, constipation, pelvic and back pain
- Most feared complication(s): Uterine necrosis, infection leading to death
- Expected outcome: Improvement in bleeding, bulk symptoms

Pre-Procedure
Indications
- Severe menstrual bleeding – flooding, anemia
- Urinary frequency, constipation, pelvic and back pain

Contraindications
- Asymptomatic fibroids, pregnancy, pelvic infection, pedunculated fibroid on thin, long stalk (serosal or submucosal), perhaps adenomyosis

Getting Started
- Things to Check
  - o Office visit with patient for history/physical, explain procedure
  - o Imaging studies demonstrating fibroids
    - ▪ US - screening
    - ▪ MRI - better definition of fibroids, evaluate for adenomyosis
  - o Normal recent pap smear; endometrial biopsy, if abnormal bleeding
- Equipment List
  - o Foley catheter
  - o One wall needle for puncture, 5 Fr sheath, Terumo glidewire
  - o Catheters
    - ▪ Omni flush for pelvic arteriogram, long reverse curve catheter
    - ▪ Alternative - Cobra catheter, microcatheters, microwires
  - o Embolization materials

Uterine Artery Embolization

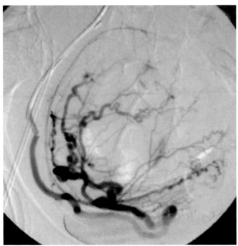

Catheter in the uterine artery placed distal to cervical artery branch. Particles being injected through catheter, preferentially go to hypervascular areas.

- ▪ PVA 300-500µ, Biospheres 500-700µ, 700-900µ, 900µ+, don't use particles smaller than 500µ, for this procedure; Gelfoam has been used, but particles are more commonly used
- ▪ Syringes 10 cc, 1 cc and 3-way stopcock for mixing particles
- o Medications: Conscious sedation, PCA for pain control; Scopolamine patch 1.5 mg to decrease nausea, nitroglycerine 100-200µg intra-arterial into uterine artery, prophylactic antibiotics –Ancef 1 gm

Procedure
Patient Position/Location
- Angiographic room, prep both groins, start on right

Procedure Steps
- Place sheath, Omni flush-catheter in aorta, level of renal arteries
- Injection in aorta, but film pelvis, allows visualization of ovarian arteries
- Reposition catheter at bifurcation, Terumo wire into left femoral artery
- Advance long reverse curve catheter until marking band at bifurcation, remove wire, advance catheter at groin, reforming reverse curve
- Catheter advanced until tip of catheter at left internal iliac artery
- Catheter pulled down, with use of contrast injections, negotiated into left internal iliac artery, then anterior division, then into uterine artery
- Hand injection, filming, verify catheter past cervical artery branch
- 200 µg of nitroglycerine via catheter helps minimize spasm
- Embolize until no flow hypervascular masses, ideally flow in main uterine artery
- Post embolization angiogram
- Reposition catheter into right uterine artery, repeat above process
- Catheter repositioned over the bifurcation, straightened and removed
- Alternative procedure: Cobra catheter, place over bifurcation, into left uterine artery, roadmapping helpful, may need microcatheters and wires
- Cobra formed into Waltman loop to catheterize the right uterine artery

Uterine Artery Embolization

Alternative Procedures/Therapies
- Surgical
  - Myomectomy
  - Hysterectomy
  - Hysteroscopic myomectomy
- Other
  - Drug therapy - non-steroidal anti-inflammatory drugs, birth-control pills, hormonal therapy

Post-Procedure
Things to Do
- Patient usually hospitalized overnight
- Pain control most important - PCA pump, NSAIDs, antiemetics
- Discharge with narcotics, NSAIDs
- Following discharge, patient needs to be alert for fever, chills, foul smelling discharge, increasing pain, may indicate uterine infection
- Return office visit 3-4 weeks, and 6 months, repeat MRI in 6 months

Things to Avoid
- Nothing per vagina for 3 weeks – help avoid infection

Common Problems & Complications
Problems
- Difficulty catheterizing uterine artery
  - Roadmapping, microcatheters, microwires
  - Approach via other groin
- Large ovarian arteries supplying fibroid
  - May embolize – possible increased risk of ovarian failure
  - Patient should be consented ahead of time for this possibility

Complications
- Severe
  - Uterine infection – requiring hysterectomy, uterine rupture
  - Pulmonary embolus
  - Unrecognized leiomyosarcoma delaying definitive treatment
- Other complications
  - Pain requiring re-hospitalization
  - Fibroid expulsion, may require D&C for treatment
  - Ovarian failure – amenorrhea and menopausal symptoms
  - Failure of procedure to correct symptoms

Selected References
1. Spies JB et al: Leiomyomata treated with uterine artery embolization: Factors associated with successful symptom and imaging outcome. Radiology 222:45-52, 2002
2. Watson GM et al: Uterine artery embolization for the treatment of symptomatic fibroids in 114 women: Reduction in size of fibroids and women's views of success of treatment. BJOG 109:129-35, 2002
3. Goodwin SC et al: Uterine artery embolization for the treatment of uterine leiomyomata midterm results. JVIR 10:1159-65, 1999

Ultrasound Puncture Femoral Artery

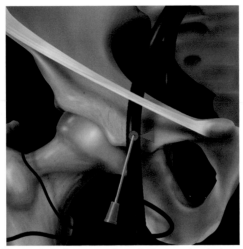

The target site for common femoral artery puncture is shown.

Key Facts
- Right common femoral artery (RCFA) is first choice site of entry for most angiography procedures
- Enables precise choice of site to puncture artery
  - RCFA bifurcation can be seen and puncture made above this level
- Ultrasound (U/S) enables frontwalling of artery reliably
- In a patient that will need thrombolysis, it is reassuring to confidently enter artery on first pass with a single wall puncture
- Enables access to arteries and grafts which lack a palpable pulse
- Ultrasound can be used to first confirm artery is patent
- Decreases patient pain by usually enabling access on first needle stick
- Enables identification of native artery versus graft which is useful when doing RCFA puncture in patient with a bypass graft

Pre-Procedure
Indications
- RCFA puncture
- Difficult to palpate artery
- Planned thrombolysis

Contraindications
- Occluded artery

Getting Started
- Things to Check
  - Check patient symptoms and labs
- Equipment List
  - Ultrasound transducer cover
  - Lidocaine with 30-gauge needle
  - #11 scalpel
  - Single wall (no stylet) or double wall (with stylet) 18-gauge needle
  - 3 mm J tip guidewire

Ultrasound Puncture Femoral Artery

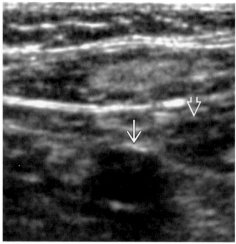

White arrow points to RCFA. Open arrow points to where RCFV is compressed. Note: RCFA put in center of FOV with maximal magnification. 2D gain remains dark to improve visualization of needle tip.

Procedure

Fluoroscopic Target Site for RCFA Entry

- Best site to enter is junction of mid and lower thirds of femoral head
- Helps ensure entry into RCFA below inguinal ligament and above RCFA bifurcation

Typical Sequence of Steps

- A hemostat is placed over site of RCFA pulse
- Location relative to femoral head confirmed with fluoroscopy

Ultrasound

- Scan RCFA and identify bifurcation
  - Puncture above this
- Ultrasound is first used to confirm RCFA is patent
- RCFA is located laterally, pulsatile, noncompressible and has a relatively thick wall
- Vein is medial, nonpulsatile, compressible and thin walled
- Local anesthetic is given to make a skin wheal on both sides of RCFA and anterior to artery
- With U/S guided arterial puncture, it is helpful to use U/S guidance for giving local anesthetic (LA) down to and around vascular structure to be punctured
  - Application of LA in this way enables less reliance on IV sedation for prevention of pain
  - This is relevant because without U/S guidance LA may mask pulse
- A small nick is made in skin with a #11 scalpel
- Nick is bluntly dissected a short distance downward with tip of hemostat
- Rationale for this dissection is that if bleeding occurs, will occur outward rather than as an occult hematoma
- Transducer is placed transverse relative to RCFA and needle is visualized as advanced into artery

- o Decrease field of view depth as much as possible to magnify size of RCFA
- o A bigger target is easier to hit
- Can use single or double wall 18 G needle or a 21 G micropuncture needle
- Put artery in center of transducer field of view
  - o Then put needle along center of transducer
  - o Maintaining this alignment will facilitate arterial entry
- Try to visualize needle from skin entry down to RCFA
  - o This works much better than trying to find needle after it has already been advanced inward
  - o Needle tip is echogenic
  - o Turning down the 2D gain will increase visibility of needle tip
- Try to puncture center of artery
  - o Works better for guidewire advancement than when side of artery is punctured
- Pulsatile blood return is observed and then guidewire is advanced into vessel

Post-Procedure
Things to Do
- Obtain hemostasis and monitor patient

Common Problems & Complications
Complications
- Dissection
- Hematoma
- Pseudoaneurysm
- Arteriovenous fistula
- Thrombosis of femoral or iliac artery

Selected References
1. Moran CJ et al: Randomized controlled trial of sheaths in diagnostic neuroangiography. RJ 218:183-7, 2001
2. Spies JB et al: Complications of femoral artery puncture. AJR 170:9-11, 1998
3. Quint LE et al: Role of femoral vessel catheterization and altered hemostasis in the development of extraperitoneal hematomas: CT study in 44 patients. AJR 160:855-8, 1993

Upper Extremity Arteriography

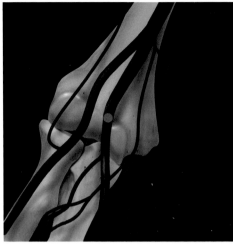

Illustration shows normal variant high/proximal origin of radial artery. If catheter tip is distal to radial artery origin, e.g. at site of yellow circle, then radial artery will not be opacified.

Key Facts
- Most common indications for upper extremity arteriography (UEA) are ischemia, trauma and as part of a dialysis graft thrombolysis procedure
- Two most common pitfalls of UEA are vasospasm, and nonvisualization of forearm and hand vessels due to normal variants

Pre-Procedure
<u>Indications</u>
- Ischemia of forearm and hand
- Trauma with potential for vascular injury
- As part of dialysis graft thrombolysis procedure

<u>Contraindications</u>
- Uncorrectable bleeding diathesis

<u>Getting Started</u>
- Things to Check
  - History of any surgery or trauma to upper extremity (UE)
  - Check if there is a history of atrial fibrillation or other arrhythmia which may have caused an embolus to UE
    - Check INR, PTT, platelets, creatinine
  - Check pulses and or doppler signal in UE to document baseline
- Equipment List
  - 5 French, 100 cm long, pigtail catheter
  - 3 mm J-tip, 145 cm long guidewire
  - Have a 200 cm, 1.5 mm J-tip wire available
  - 0.035" angled tip, 150 cm long glidewire
  - 5 French, 100 cm long, hockey-tip-type catheter
  - Nitroglycerin at a concentration of 100 micrograms/cc
  - Visipaque contrast

Upper Extremity Arteriography

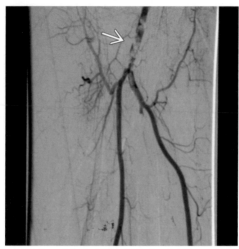

Filling defect represents embolus to left brachial artery (white arrow) in elderly patient with atrial fibrillation who presented with ischemia of the hand. Note: Prominent collateral vessels.

Procedure

Patient Position
- Supine with hand supinated in anatomic position
  - Often helpful to tape it in position
  - Tape securely enough to remind patient not to move, but not so tight as to compress vessels

Usual Sequence of Steps
- Place 5 French sheath in right femoral artery
- Place a pigtail catheter in thoracic aorta just proximal to origin of innominate artery
  - Obtain a thoracic aortogram with LAO view
- Catheterize subclavian artery with hockey tip catheter
- 0.035" angled-tip glidewire may be needed to get hockey tip catheter to go into subclavian artery
- May then need a 3 mm J-tip guidewire to advance further into subclavian or axillary artery
  - Benefit is its bulky tip tends to stay in subclavian and axillary arteries and not go into small side branches as a glidewire has a tendency to do
- Keep hand warm throughout procedure
  - Can cover hand with a warm towel
  - Coldness causes vasospasm

Upper Arm Arteriogram
- Obtain arteriogram of upper arm with catheter in proximal axillary artery
- Will facilitate detection of variants such as high origin of radial or ulnar artery
- Use Visipaque contrast which is nonionic and less likely to cause discomfort and patient motion

Forearm and Hand Arteriogram
- Advance catheter into brachial artery

Upper Extremity Arteriography

- Can administer 100-200 micrograms of NTG intra-arterially
  - Helps to optimize vasodilation
- Obtain arteriogram of forearm and hand
- Unless high origin of radial or ulnar artery, then advance catheter into distal brachial artery to obtain magnified arteriogram of hand
- Obtain magnified AP view arteriogram of hand
- Try to avoid entering radial or ulnar arteries as may develop pericatheter vasospasm and thrombosis

Normal Variants
- Aberrant right and left subclavian artery are rare
- Left vertebral artery origin directly from arch is also rare
- High origin of radial artery in approximately 15%
- High origin of ulnar artery in approximately 2%
- Common interosseus artery from proximal brachial artery
- Duplication of brachial artery is rare
- Variations of deep and superficial palmar arches

Causes of UE Ischemia
- Atherosclerotic narrowing of subclavian artery is most common lesion in elderly persons
  - May cause subclavian steal syndrome
- Thoracic outlet syndrome with formation of aneurysm
  - Can lead to distal embolization from thrombus in aneurysm
- Embolus from heart
  - Causes include atrial fibrillation, old infarction with ventricular aneurysm, and prosthetic valves
- Dialysis graft with "steal" of arterial flow away from hand
- Trauma
- Diabetes
- Raynaud's disease
- Buerger's disease

Post-Procedure

Things to Do
- Obtain hemostasis and monitor patient

Common Problems & Complications

- Vasospasm
- Arterial thrombosis
- Dissection
- Stroke
- Puncture site complications
- Misdiagnosis due to a failure to detect a normal variant such as a high origin of radial or ulnar artery

Selected References
1. Johnson SP et al: Acute arterial occlusions of the small vessels of the hand and forearm: Treatment with regional urokinase therapy. JVIR 10:869-76, 1999
2. Lambiase RE et al: Treatment of upper extremity thromboembolic disease with urokinase. JVIR 4:698, 1993
3. Pallan TM et al: Incompatibility of Isovue 370 and papaverine in peripheral arteriography. Radiology 187:257-9, 1993

PocketRadiologist™
Interventional
Top 100 Procedures

NEUROANGIOGRAPHY

Cerebral Angiography Basics

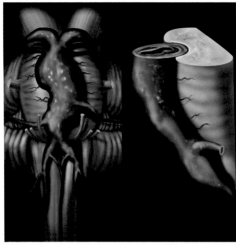

Graphic depicts atherosclerotic fusiform aneurysm of the vertebrobasilar system.

Key Facts
- Discuss indication and goals of procedure with referral service
- Check all procedure equipment available and ready before start procedure

Pre-Procedure

Indications
- Carotid stenosis, subarachnoid hemorrhage, aneurysm, AVM, vasculitis

Contraindications
- Same information readily available with less invasive test

Getting Started
- Things to Check
  - Bleeding history, platelets, PT, PTT, INR, creatinine
  - History of any previous ultrasounds, CTA, MRA or cerebral arteriograms
  - History of vascular disease related to puncture site and aorta
  - Write a pre-procedure note
- Equipment List
  - 5 French (Fr) sheath and 3-0 monofilament nylon suture
  - Flow switch (a simpler alternative than using a stopcock)
  - Pigtail catheter for thoracic aorta
  - Hockey-stick tip catheters for right carotid (Ca) and vertebral arteries (Va)
    - E.g. Berenstein and Davis are hockey-stick tip catheters
    - If use Berenstein, use braided version for better torque control
    - Simmons #3 catheter is very helpful for selecting left common carotid artery (LCCA) when has retrograde origin
  - 0.038" diameter, long tip glidewire
  - Heparinized saline flush solution in pressure bag and flush bag
  - Color coded syringes for local anesthetic, contrast and saline flush
    - Having more contrast and flush syringes decreases time used for refilling syringes during procedure

Cerebral Angiography Basics

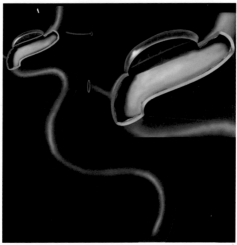

Graphic depicts a blood blisterlike aneurysm arising along the greater curvature of the supraclinoid ICA. The aneurysm wall consists of a thin, fibrous cap.

Procedure

Patient Position
- Supine

Equipment Preparation
- Flush sheath, catheter and glidewire
- Withdraw 3 to 4 cc of air into each syringe to make a big bubble
- Let smaller bubbles coalesce into this bubble
- Turn syringe on side so bubbles have shorter distance to go to coalesce
- Connect sidearm of sheath to heparinized saline pressure bag

Procedure Steps
- Obtain access to right common femoral artery and place 5 Fr sheath
- Suture sheath to skin with 3-0 monofilament nylon
- This helps to avoid complete inadvertent removal of sheath
- Also prevents intermittent partial withdrawal of sheath which can interfere with selective catheterization
- Use pigtail catheter to obtain thoracic arch arteriogram
- Evaluate arch to choose catheters for catheterization of Ca and Va
- Perform catheterizations and obtain at least 2 views of each area
- Learn to set up views quickly
- Always do hand injection to assess a vessel, prior to doing a power injector injection, to avoid overinjecting a hypoplastic, dissected or occluded vessel
- Typical views of cervical portion of internal carotid artery (ICa) are ipsilateral oblique, posteroanterior (PA) and lateral
- Typical views of intracranial portion of ICa are PA and lateral
  - Orbital roofs are superimposed on petrous ridges on PA view
- Typical views of intracranial portion of Va are PA Towne and lateral

Working with Sheaths
- "Numbering" of a sheath denotes diameter of catheter it allows
  - E.g. a 5 Fr sheath allows passage of a 5 Fr catheter
- Outer diameter ("OD") of a sheath is, of course, larger than inner

- E.g. "OD" of a 5 Fr sheath is about 6.4 Fr
- 3 Fr=1 mm
- Therefore 6 Fr=2mm
- For most procedures, a short sheath is used which is about 10 cm long
  - When iliac artery is tortuous and difficult to traverse, then may be preferable to use 25 cm long sheath
- Helpful to give local anesthetic (LA) for suture placement at same time LA given for arterial puncture
- When suture sheath, tie first knot snug to skin to minimize play in sheath
  - Make at least one square knot to secure suture to skin
  - Then pass suture thru plastic suture hole on sheath hub
    - Now tie at least 3 knots
- Sheath sidearm is connected to pressure bag which is pumped up to 300 mm Hg so that bag pressure is higher than systemic arterial pressure
  - Dial on manometer of pressure bag shows pressure
- If pressure in bag drops below 300 mm Hg during procedure, then ask technologist or nurse to pump up bag again

Syringes and Double Flush Technique
- Syringes should be cleared of air bubbles
  - Air bubble emboli can cause ischemic stroke
  - "No bubbles, no troubles"
- Double flush technique involves aspiration of catheter contents with 1st syringe followed by locking with heparinized saline from 2nd syringe
  - "Flick" or tap syringe #2 with fingers when connect to catheter to clear bubbles at site where connect to catheter
  - Hold syringe #2 upright so bubbles move away from catheter
  - Make sure to close flow switch while injecting flush solution
  - Common mistake is to stop injecting flush solution and then to clamp flow switch, which allows reflux of blood back into catheter tip

Working with Catheters and Glidewires
- Ca and especially Va are prone to spasm
  - Important to be gentle with catheter
- Keep glidewire wet so remains slippery and passes thru catheter quickly
- Standards of cleanliness are higher for cerebral angiography than peripheral angiography
  - A tiny blood clot inadvertently injected could cause an ischemic stroke
  - Try to keep catheters, syringes and procedure table free of blood clot
  - Sterile towels can be placed on top of blood that gets on table

Post-Procedure
- Observe patient 3 to 6 hours without moving leg on side of puncture

Common Problems & Complications
- Puncture site complications
- Spasm of Va or less commonly of ICa
- Ischemic stroke

Selected References
1. Randoux B et al: Carotid artery stenosis: Prospective comparison of CT, three-dimensional Gadolinium-enhanced MR, and conventional angiography. Radiology 220:179-85, 2001
2. Wolpert SM et al: Current role of cerebral angiography in the diagnosis of cerebrovascular diseases. AJR 159:191-7, 1992
3. Caplan LR et al: Angiography in patients with occlusive cerebrovascular disease: Views of a stroke neurologist and neuroradiologist. AJNR 12:593-601, 1991

Aneurysm Coiling

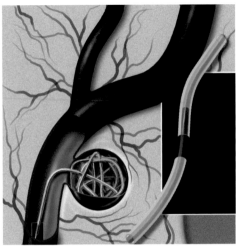

Illustration showing a microcatheter and coil placed within an aneurysm. The inset demonstrates proper alignment of the coil marker (gray) and the proximal microcatheter marker (black) prior to detachment.

Key Facts
- Procedure definition: Coil embolization of intracranial aneurysms
- Clinical setting triggering procedure: Intracranial aneurysm
- Best procedure approach: Transfemoral guide catheter placed in ICA with subsequent intra-aneurysmal microcatheter placement & coil embolization
- Most feared complications
  - Aneurysm rupture
  - Embolic stroke
  - Branch vessel occlusion
  - Coil prolapse into parent vessel
- Expected outcome: Exclusion of aneurysm from cerebral circulation

Pre-Procedure
Indications
- Clinical setting triggering procedure: Ruptured or unruptured intracranial aneurysm with suitable aneurysm neck geometry & lack of incorporation of parent vessel branches
  - Anterior communicating, basilar tip, & paraclinoid aneurysms particularly suitable due to difficult surgical exposure
  - MCA aneurysms often more suitable for clipping due to surgical accessibility & frequent incorporation of parent vessel branches
Contraindications
- Unfavorable aneurysm geometry/location
- Inability to access aneurysm due to proximal vascular occlusion
- Renal failure (relative)
- Uncorrected coagulopathy (relative)
Getting Started
- Things to Check
  - Imaging studies (CT, MR, & prior angio)

Aneurysm Coiling

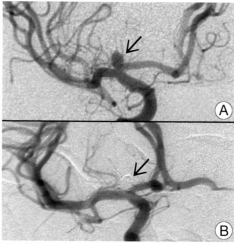

Unruptured right ICA terminus aneurysm. (A) narrow-necked spherical aneurysm arising from ICA bifurcation (arrow) was discovered on MRI in this 61 year-old female. (B) The aneurysm was successfully treated with four coils (arrow).

- Ventriculostomy catheter to be placed prior to coiling in patients with ruptured aneurysms & ventriculomegaly
- Ventriculostomy kit should be in room (readily available)
  - BUN, creatinine, PT, PTT, INR
  - Availability of anesthesia (most cases are performed under general)
- Medications
  - Unruptured aneurysms: Clopidogrel (Plavix) 75 mg & aspirin 325 mg daily commencing 4 days prior to procedure
- Equipment List
  - High quality angiography machine with biplane fluoroscopy
  - 6 Fr sheath, 5 Fr neuroangiocatheter & a 0.035" angled-tip glidewire
  - 2 rotating hemostatic valves (RHV)
  - 5 or 6 Fr guiding catheter (Envoy, Cordis; or Guider, Target)
  - 0.038" extra stiff exchange wire (Extra Stiff Amplatz Wire; Cook, Inc.)
  - Microcatheter with proximal (3 cm from tip) & distal markers
    - 0.010" coil compatible (Excelsior-SL10, Target; Prowler 10 or 14, Cordis)
    - 0.018" coil compatible (Excelsior-1018, Target; Prowler Plus, Cordis)
  - 0.010" or 0.014" microwire (Synchro, Precision Vascular; Transend, Target; or Agility, Cordis)
  - 0.010" or 0.018" detachable coils (10 coils for aneurysms < 10 mm)
    - 3D framing coils (Target, Micrus, MicroVention or Cordis)
    - Non-3D filling coils (Target, Micrus, MicroVention or Cordis)

Procedure
Patient Position/Location
- Angio suite with patient supine
- Radiopaque marker is placed on head for measurements

Aneurysm Coiling

Equipment Preparation
- Flush all catheters/sheaths
- Activate hydrophilic coating on catheters/wires by immersion in saline

Procedure Steps
- Patient under general anesthesia & Foley inserted
- Access femoral artery & perform baseline angiogram
  - Measure aneurysm & select working view which optimally shows relationship of aneurysm neck to parent vessel
- Heparinize (ACT twice baseline) if unruptured aneurysm
- Ruptured aneurysm: Heparinize after first coil is placed or not at all
- Select ECA on side to be treated with glidewire & 5 Fr catheter
- Anchor a 0.038" extra stiff exchange wire in ECA & exchange for the 5 or 6 Fr guiding catheter which is placed below bifurcation
- Select & advance guide to level of distal cervical ICA & attach RHV with heparinized/pressurized saline drip
- Roadmap image obtained in working view
- Insert microcatheter/wire (attached to RHV with heparinized/pressurized saline drip) & place tip of microwire in aneurysm & then carefully advance microcatheter into aneurysm
  - Tip of catheter should be near center of aneurysm – if tip is against wall may rupture aneurysm when coil is placed
- Place appropriate diameter/length 3D framing coil & perform angiogram
  - If angiogram shows no coil prolapse then electrolytically (Target, Micrus) or hydrostatically (MicroVention, Cordis) detach coil
- Aneurysm is then filled with increasingly smaller filling coils
  - After the 3D coil is placed subsequent coils can be placed using a roadmap performed without contrast to subtract-out initial coil mass
- Final intracranial angio to exclude embolic complication
- Heparin discontinued & sheath removed when ACT < 180 (or closure device is used)

Alternative Procedures/Therapies
- Surgical: Clipping

Post-Procedure
- Admit to ICU with close monitoring of neuro status & BP
- IV fluids (NS)
- Plavix x 6 weeks & aspirin for life in coiled unruptured aneurysms
- F/U angio at 6 & 12 months to exclude regrowth

Common Problems & Complications
Problems
- Wide-necked aneurysms may require balloon/stent assisted technique

Complications
- Stroke (GP IIb/IIIa inhibitors useful in unruptured aneurysms)
- Aneurysm rupture (have protamine sulfate available & be prepared to rapidly place additional coils)

Selected References
1. Cloft HJ et al: Use of three-dimensional guglielmi detachable coils in the treatment of wide-necked cerebral aneurysms. AJNR 21:1312-4, 2000
2. Vinuela F et al: Guglielmi detachable coil embolization of acute intracranial aneurysm: perioperative anatomical and clinical outcome in 403 patients. Neurosurgery 86:457-82, 1997
3. Guglielmi G et al: Electrothrombosis of saccular aneurysms via endovascular approach. Neurosurgery 75:1-7, 1991

Angioplasty for Vasospasm

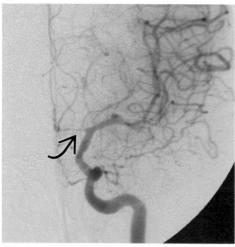

AP view left ICA angiogram in a patient who is six days status post basilar artery tip aneurysm rupture & clipping. There is significant spasm involving A1 segment of left ACA (curved arrow). Correlation with the initial angiogram to exclude a hypoplastic A1 is necessary (dilatation of which may result in vessel rupture).

Key Facts
- Procedure definition: Percutaneous transluminal angioplasty (PTA) for vasospasm
  - Vasospasm is leading cause of disability & death after intracranial aneurysm rupture
- Clinical setting triggering procedure: Symptomatic vasospasm (progressive neurologic deficits) 2° to subarachnoid hemorrhage
  - Vasospasm usually begins on day 3, maximal at 6-8 days & resolves around 12th day following SAH
- Best procedure approach: Compliant balloon for PTA of ICA, vertebro-basilar arteries, M1 and A1 arteries
- Most feared complication(s): Vessel rupture & reperfusion hemorrhage of infarcted areas (rare)
- Expected outcome: Restoration of vessel diameter & blood flow

Pre-Procedure
Indications
- Symptomatic vasospasm 2° to subarachnoid hemorrhage
  - Refractory to medical therapy
    - Triple H therapy: Hemodilution, hypertension, & hypervolemia
    - Calcium antagonists: Nimodipine (60 mg q 4 hrs x 21 days)
  - Often used in conjunction with papaverine infusion (for distal vessels unreachable with PTA)
Contraindications
- Large region(s) of infarction/hemorrhage
Getting Started
- Things to Check
  - Prior angiogram to assess pre-vasospasm appearance of vessels

Angioplasty for Vasospasm

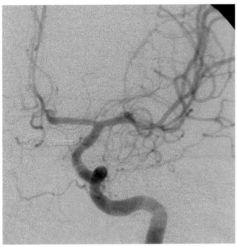

Post angioplasty image shows marked improvement in the diameter of the A1 segment of the ACA. A Sentry OTW balloon catheter was used to gain access to the ACA (case courtesy E.A. Stevens, MD).

- It is imperative not to mistakenly treat a vessel that is hypoplastic rather than spastic due to risk of rupture
  o Patient's neurologic status to predict involved vascular territories
  o Transcranial doppler (TCD) velocities
    - A sudden increase in TCD > 120 cm/sec or MCA/ICA ratio of > 3 correlate with onset of vasospasm (> 6 = severe spasm)
  o CT for infarction, hemorrhage or hydrocephalus
  o Availability of anesthesia
  o BUN, creatinine, PT, PTT, INR
- Equipment List
  o Angiography suite
  o 5 French neuroangiography catheter & 0.035" angled-tip glidewire
  o 6 French guiding catheter
  o Rotating hemostatic valve (RHV)
  o Compliant angioplasty balloons
    - Flow-directed: Endeavor (Target) nondetachable silicone balloon
    - Over-the-wire (OTW): Sentry (Target), Commodore (Cordis), Hyperglide (MTI)

Procedure

Procedure Steps
- Access femoral artery & perform diagnostic angiogram
  o Assess presence & extent of vasospasm
- Prep balloon with 50% contrast
  o Air bubbles diffuse through silicone (inflate & leave on table 5 - 10 min)
  o Endeavor: 0.010" wire (placed through an RHV) used for support & advanced up to level of balloon
  o OTW systems prepped with an RHV & appropriate wire
  o 1 cc syringe & flow-switch/stopcock attached to RHV for inflations

Angioplasty for Vasospasm

- Treat most symptomatic side first by accessing external carotid with exchange glidewire & advancing guiding catheter into common carotid, then select ICA & place guide catheter in distal cervical ICA
  - ICA is prone to spasm in these patients & hyperdynamic state (guide catheter motion) can predispose to dissection
- A decision is made whether to heparinize & if heparin is used the target ACT by bolus & infusion is twice baseline
- ICA vasospasm
  - Lateral roadmap & endeavor balloon
  - Test inflation performed in cavernous segment
  - Endeavor is advanced to level of vasospasm & a series of at least 4 short sequential inflations performed (25%, 50%, 75% & 100% of original vessel diameter)
  - Balloon is moved distally & sequence is repeated
- MCA, vertebrobasilar, & PCA vasospasm
  - Same technique as ICA but with AP roadmap
  - Usually limit PTA to proximal MCA (M1) & PCA (P1)
- ACA vasospasm
  - Flow-guided balloon accesses ACA < 10% of time
    - Collateral flow after ICA & MCA PTA may be sufficient, if PTA is performed an OTW balloon is often needed

Post-Procedure
Things to Do
- Patient is returned to neuro intensive care & frequent neuro checks are performed

Common Problems & Complications
Problems
- Must not inadvertently enter small branch vessels (e.g. PComA, AChA, or PICA) due to risk of rupture with inflation
  - Good roadmap mandatory: Low threshold for general anesthesia
- May be difficult to dilate focal spasm with flow-guided balloon due to watermelon seeding
  - Use OTW system (more stable) if necessary
- Unable to access ACA: Assess collateral flow & determine necessity
  - If necessary use OTW system or infuse papaverine with intermittent balloon occlusion of MCA with Endeavor
- Supplement distal or inaccessible vasospasm with papaverine infusion
Complications
- Severe
  - 5–10% risk of stroke or death
  - Reperfusion hemorrhage (rare)
  - Vessel rupture: Usually due to dilatation of small branch vessel

Selected References
1. Smith TP et al: Endovascular treatment of cerebral vasospasm. JVIR 11:547-59, 2000
2. Eskridge JM: A practical approach to the treatment of vasospasm. AJNR 18:1653-60, 1997
3. Barnwell SL et al: Transluminal angioplasty of intracerebral vessels for cerebral arterial spasm: reversal of neurological deficits after delayed treatment. Neurosurgery 25:424-9, 1989

Carotid Angiography Head

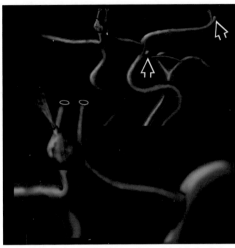

Graphic depiction of the circle of Willis shows a large, lobulated, aCoA aneurysm with rupture into the subarachnoid space. Unruptured aneurysms are also depicted at the MCA and PCoA (open arrows).

Key Facts
- Discuss indication and goals of procedure with referral service
- Tailor the study to answer the clinical question
- Catheterize main artery of interest first
- Embolic stroke and aneurysm rupture are most feared complications

Pre-Procedure
Indications
- Subarachnoid hemorrhage (SAH) and vasospasm are most common urgent indications
- Carotid stenosis and intracranial arterial stenosis
- AVM and cerebral vasculitis
- Acute ischemic stroke in candidates for transcatheter thrombolysis
- Preoperative evaluation of tumors such as large meningiomas to determine vascular supply, check for venous sinus thrombosis and for endovascular embolization

Contraindications
- Same information readily available with less invasive test

Getting Started
- Things to Check
  o Bleeding history, platelets, PT, PTT, INR, creatinine
  o History of previous ultrasounds, CTA, MRA or arteriograms
  o History of vascular disease related to puncture site and aorta
  o Write a pre-procedure note
- Equipment List
  o Please see other chapters on carotid and vertebral angiography

Procedure
Patient Position
- Supine

Carotid Angiography Head

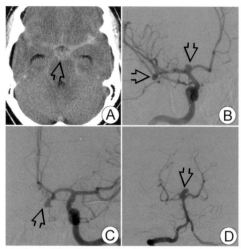

(A) CECT scan shows diffuse SAH. (B, C, D) DSA shows multiple small aneurysms (arrows). The large, irregular, ACoA aneurysm (C, arrow) is the one that ruptured.

Equipment Preparation
- Flush sheath, catheter and glidewire
- Make sure contrast and heparin flush syringes are free of bubbles

Anatomy
- There are several different classifications of ICA anatomy
- One useful way to describe ICA segments is as follows: Cervical, ascending petrous, horizontal petrous, precavernous, cavernous and supraclinoid which then bifurcates into ACA and MCA
- Anterior cerebral artery (ACA) segments are labeled A1, A2, A3, and A4
  - Anterior communicating artery connects right and left A1-A2 junctions
- Middle cerebral artery (MCA) segments are labeled M1, M2, M3, and M4

Procedure Steps
- Place catheter into common carotid (CCA) or internal carotid artery (ICA)
- Advantages of CCA catheter position are easier to select, usually works well for most indications and less risk of spasm
- Advantages of ICA position are avoid overlap of ECA branches, catheter less likely to kick out, and critically ill patients less likely to move during injection because avoid discomfort of contrast injection into ECA

Selecting Internal Carotid Artery
- Any hockey-tip catheter can be used
- CCA bifurcation (CCAB) is shaped similarly to letter "U" with ECA anterior and ICA posterior
- Always do hand injection of contrast with catheter in CCA to assess CCAB before crossing it with guide wire and catheter
- Roadmap angiography in lateral projection is helpful for selecting ICA
- If ICA widely patent, then simply direct tip of catheter posteriorly and advance over guidewire into ICA
- Some angiographers may use hand injection "puffs" of contrast to serve as a "hydrostatic guide wire"
- Try to position catheter tip in ICA parallel to long axis of vessel
- A typical injection rate with ICA catheter is 4 cc per second for 6 cc total

Carotid Angiography Head

Routine Views
- For posterior-anterior view, superimpose orbital roofs on petrous ridges
  o Improves visualization of ICA bifurcation, ACA and MCA
- For lateral view, try to superimpose orbital roofs and external ears

Additional Views
- Angiographers should also be familiar with Towne, Waters, transorbital oblique and submental vertex views

Subarachnoid Hemorrhage
- Evaluate CT scan to help determine likely site of aneurysm
- Goal is to delineate aneurysm size, orientation, relationship to parent vessel and adjacent branches
  o A coin such as a USA dime placed anterior, posterior and on both sides of head can be helpful for measurement of aneurysms
  o A dime measures 18 mm in diameter
  o Some angiography machines have useful built-in measuring capabilities
- Important to try to clearly show aneurysm neck
  o May require multiple oblique views and a magnified view
  o Fast film rates can help differentiate vascular loop from aneurysm
  o Rotational angiography helpful
- Additional goal is to detect multiple aneurysms
  o Complete study includes carotid and vertebrobasilar territory with visualization of anterior communicating artery and bilateral posterior inferior cerebellar arteries
- Check collateral circulation and for any branches arising from aneurysm dome
- Multiple aneurysms are present in approximately 20%
  o Findings to suggest likely source of bleeding include larger size, irregular shape, and larger amount of adjacent blood on CT scan
- If all injections were made in ICA and do not find an aneurysm, then do an injection with catheter in CCA as may reveal another cause of bleeding such as a dural arteriovenous fistula (DAVF)
- Differential diagnosis of SAH with negative arteriogram includes benign perimesencephalic hemorrhage, incomplete arteriogram, posttraumatic SAH, thrombosed aneurysm, blister aneurysm, DAVF and tumor
- Performance of thoracic aorta arch angiography is helpful in older patients as origins of great vessels may be narrowed, and tortuous anatomy may affect choice of guiding catheter for endovascular therapy

Post-Procedure
- Observe patient 3 to 6 hours without moving leg on side of puncture

Common Problems & Complications
- Puncture site complications
- Spasm, dissection and ischemic stroke

Selected References
1. Randoux B et al: Carotid artery stenosis: Prospective comparison of CT, three-dimensional Gadolinium-enhanced MR, and conventional angiography. Radiology 220:179-85, 2001
2. Wolpert SM et al: Current role of cerebral angiography in the diagnosis of cerebrovascular diseases. AJR 159:191-7, 1992
3. Caplan LR et al: Angiography in patients with occlusive cerebrovascular disease: views of a stroke neurologist and neuroradiologist. AJNR 12:593-601, 1991

Carotid Angiography Neck

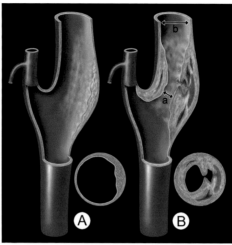

Graphic depiction of mild and severe carotid atherosclerosis (ASVD). (A) Earliest signs of ASVD are "fatty streaks" and slight intimal thickening. (B) Severe stenosis with intraplaque hemorrhage, ulceration and platelet emboli are shown. NASCET calculation % stenosis=b-a/b x 100.

Key Facts
- Most common indication is preoperative evaluation of carotid stenosis
- Try to selectively catheterize main artery of interest first
- Ipsilateral oblique is usually best view to minimize overlap of internal carotid (ICA) and external carotid (ECA) arteries
- Embolic stroke is most severe complication

Pre-Procedure
Indications
- Carotid ultrasound (U/S), CTA or MRA suggestive of occlusion
  - Angiography can show occlusion more accurately than U/S
  - High-grade stenoses are often treated with surgery, whereas occlusions are usually managed nonoperatively
- Long segment stenosis of ICA, to determine if amenable to standard surgery or if extends above jaw and less amenable to surgery
- As part of cerebral arteriogram where main focus is intracranial
  - Images of neck vessels may help for treatment planning
- Carotid angioplasty and stenting
- Neck trauma
Contraindications
- Same information readily available with less invasive test
Getting Started
- Things to Check
  - Bleeding history, platelets, PT, PTT, INR, creatinine
  - History of any previous U/S, CTA, MRA or cerebral arteriograms
  - Write a preprocedure note
- Equipment List
  - Hockey stick tip catheters for right carotid (Ca) and vertebral arteries (Va)
    - In young patients hockey tip may be used for bilateral carotids

Carotid Angiography Neck

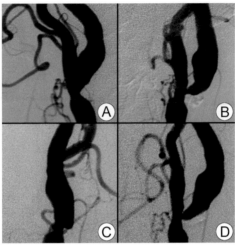

(A-D) 4 views of common carotid DSA are shown. Maximum stenosis is profiled in (B). For calculation % stenosis, see graphic in the previous page.

- o Simmons #3 catheter is helpful for selecting a left common carotid artery (LCCA) with a retrograde origin, which is common in older patients
- o 0.038" diameter, long tip glidewire
- o Connector tubing between catheter and power injector is helpful in that allows check for bubbles without drawing blood into power injector

Procedure

Patient Position
- Supine

Thoracic Aorta Arch Arteriogram (TAAA)
- Use pigtail catheter to obtain TAAA in LAO and RAO projections
- Evaluate arch to choose catheters for catheterization of carotid arteries

Selecting Right Common Carotid Artery (RCCA)
- RCCA is usually straightforward to catheterize
- Main exception is with tortuous innominate artery
  - o Guidewire may tend to go into right subclavian artery
  - o Roadmap angiography is helpful in this situation
- Advantage of hockey tip over Simmons catheter, is hockey tip catheters do not need to be formed and facilitate catheterization of ICA
  - o Hockey tip also facilitates later catheterization of vertebral artery
- Glidewire is passed into RCCA and is followed by hockey-tip catheter
- Glidewire is withdrawn, and catheter is double flushed
- For carotid stenosis angiography, catheter tip is typically positioned in proximal to mid common carotid artery
  - o This is also often adequate for cerebral aneurysm angiography, but sometimes will want to catheterize internal carotid artery
- Typical views of cervical portion of internal carotid artery are ipsilateral oblique, posteroanterior (PA) and lateral

Carotid Angiography Neck

- Try to position tip of catheter within RCCA so that orientated parallel to long axis of vessel and tip is not against vessel wall
- Hand injection is made to assess flow and is used to choose injection rate
- Typical injection rates for common carotid angiography are 5 to 8 cc per second for a total of 7 to 12 cc
  - A commonly used rate is 6 cc per second for a total of 8 cc

Selecting Left Common Carotid Artery (LCCA)
- In young patients LCCA origin is relatively straight and can usually be catheterized with a hockey tip catheter
- In older patients origin often has a steep angulation
- LCCA arising from innominate artery is referred to as a "bovine arch"
- More commonly, left carotid will arise directly from aortic arch
- Key step is to very slowly withdraw catheter from RCCA-innominate artery (R-I A)
  - If done too quickly, catheter will miss and go into left subclavian
- As catheter withdrawn, keep tip pointed upwards so will "pop" into LCCA
- Inject contrast to confirm in left carotid and then advance catheter inward until its position is secure for an angiographic filming series

Using a Simmons Catheter
- Simmons #3 has a longer tip than Simmons #1 or #2
- Some highly tortuous LCCAs can only be selected by a Simmons #2 or #3
- Simmons #3 is most common catheter used for LCCA at author's hospital
- Catheter tip is usually formed by rotation at junction of thoracic arch and descending aorta, but subclavian artery can also be used to form tip
- Tip is pointed upward in ascending aorta and catheter withdrawn to select RCCA or LCCA
- To select LCCA as exit R-IA, must turn tip anteriorly as slowly withdraw
- Simmons catheter is unique in that advancement of catheter at groin level will cause withdrawal of catheter tip
  - This is opposite of other types of angiographic catheters
- Typically catheter will now "pop" into left common carotid
- Above twisting of catheter will create a torque effect which must be relieved before catheter position will be secure
- Simply twist catheter in opposite direction so that distal loop of Simmons catheter will be opened up
- Inject contrast to confirm position in LCCA

Post-Procedure
Things to Do
- Observe patient 3 to 6 hours without moving leg on side of puncture

Common Problems & Complications
- Puncture site complications
- Knotted Simmons catheter
- Stroke due to embolus of air, thrombus or atherosclerotic debris
- Stroke due to dissection by guidewire or catheter

Selected References
1. Yousem DM et al:Injection rates for neuroangiography: Results of a survey. AJNR 22:1838-40, 2001
2. Martin MA et al: Vasa vasorum: Another cause of carotid string sign. AJNR 20:259-62, 1999
3. Heiserman JE et al: Neurologic complications of cerebral angiography. AJNR 15:1401-7, 1994

Carotid Stenting

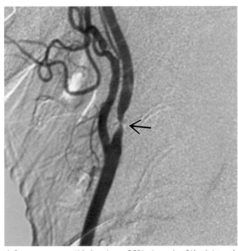

Lateral view left common carotid showing a 90% stenosis of the internal carotid 1 cm from the origin (arrow).

Key Facts
- Procedure definition: Endovascular carotid revascularization
- Clinical setting triggering procedure
  - Symptomatic carotid stenosis > 50% by North American Symptomatic Carotid Endarterectomy Trial (NASCET) criteria
  - Asymptomatic carotid stenosis > 70% by (NASCET) criteria
- Best procedure approach: Trans-femoral sheath placed in CCA with pre-dilation angioplasty & self-expanding stent placement
- Most feared complications
  - Embolic stroke
  - Bradycardia & asystole due to vagal stimulation
  - Cerebral hyperperfusion syndrome & hemorrhage
  - Acute stent thrombosis
- Expected outcome
  - < 20% residual stenosis
  - Absence of recurrent neurologic symptoms

Pre-Procedure
Indications
- Carotid artery stenting (CAS) remains investigational & usually performed in patients who are poor risk for carotid endarterectomy (CEA)
  - Significant cardiac & noncardiac comorbid conditions
  - Contralateral carotid occlusion
  - Recurrent stenosis post CEA
  - Post head & neck radiation stenosis (fibrosis)
  - High (retro-mandibular) carotid bifurcation
Contraindications
- Uncorrected coagulopathy
- Recent lobar infarction
- Angiographic evidence of thrombus at level of stenosis

Carotid Stenting

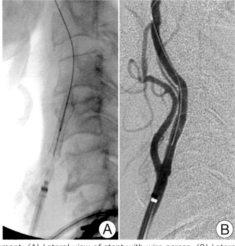

Post deployment. (A) Lateral view of stent with wire across. (B) Lateral angiogram showing an adequate initial result. A post-stenting angioplasty was not performed. An 8 X 20 mm Precise Stent (Cordis Endovascular) was used.

- Renal failure

Getting Started

- Things to Check
    - Imaging studies (CT, MR, US, & prior angio)
    - BUN, creatinine, PT, PTT, INR
- Medications
    - Aspirin 325 mg daily commencing 4 days prior to procedure
    - Clopidogrel (Plavix) 75 mg daily commencing 4 days prior to procedure
    - Glycopyrrolate (Robinul) 0.2-0.4 mg IV given prior to angioplasty to prevent bradycardia
    - Heparin 5,000 IU (maintain ACT twice baseline) prior to placing guide
    - Anti-hypertensive medications are held day of procedure
    - Hydrate with IV normal saline
- Equipment List
    - Angiography suite
    - 5 Fr sheath with pigtail & neuroangiography catheter & 0.035" angled tip glidewire
    - 7 Fr 90 cm guiding sheath (Shuttle; Cook, Inc.)
    - 0.038" extra stiff exchange wire (Extra Stiff Amplatz Wire; Cook, Inc.)
    - 0.014" exchange length microwire
    - 4 x 40 mm low profile angioplasty balloon (Savvy; Cordis Endovascular)
    - Self-expanding stent (Precise Stent; Cordis Endovascular; or Wallstent; Boston Scientific Scimed Inc.)
    - 5 or 6 x 20 mm balloon for post-dilation (use diameter of distal ICA)

Procedure

Patient Position/Location

- Angio suite with patient supine
- Radiopaque marker is placed on ipsilateral neck for measurements

Carotid Stenting

Equipment Preparation
- Flush all catheters/sheaths
- Activate hydrophilic coating on catheters/wires by immersion in saline

Procedure Steps
- Foley inserted
- Access femoral artery & perform 3 vessel angiogram
  - Assess collaterals & establish baseline appearance of intracranial vasculature
  - Measure stenosis & select stent that is 2 mm larger than largest portion of artery to be covered
    - If stent extends into CCA, this would mean a 10 mm stent in most men & 8 mm stent in most women
- Select ECA on side to be treated with glidewire & 5 Fr catheter
- Anchor a 0.038" extra stiff exchange wire in ECA & exchange for the 7 Fr 90 cm guiding sheath placed below bifurcation
- Cross stenosis with 0.014" wire & pre-dilate with 4 mm balloon
- Check angiographic result through guide
- May exchange for 0.018" wire if there is significant proximal tortuosity
- Exchange for & deploy stent & perform angiogram with wire across stent
- Assess need for post-stent angioplasty
  - < 20% residual stenosis optimal
  - Since self-expanding stents will continue to expand & most embolic events occur during post-dilation a less than optimal initial result is often acceptable
- Final cervical & intra-cranial angio to exclude embolic complication
- Heparin discontinued & sheath removed when ACT < 180 (or closure device is used)

Alternative Procedures/Therapies
- Carotid endarterectomy

Post-Procedure

Things to Do
- Admit to ICU x 24 Hrs with close monitoring of neuro status & BP
- Plavix 75 mg/day x 4–6 weeks & aspirin 325 mg/day indefinitely

Common Problems & Complications

Problems
- Acute angle origin of left CCA may require a 5 Fr 125 cm catheter (VTK Thorocon NB, Cook, Inc.) placed coaxially through guiding sheath

Complications
- Stroke (several distal protection devices currently in trials)
- Acute or delayed bradycardia (may require temporary trans-venous pacemaker &/or dopamine infusion)

Selected References
1. Kirsch EC et al: Carotid arterial stent placement: Results and follow-up in 53 patients. Radiology 220:737-44, 2001
2. Phatouros CC et al: Endovascular stenting for carotid artery stenosis: Preliminary experience using the Shape-Memory-Alloy-Recoverable-Technology (SMART) Stent. AJNR 21:732-8, 2000
3. Vitek JJ et al: Carotid artery stenting: Technical considerations. AJNR 21:1736-43, 2000

Epistaxis Embolization

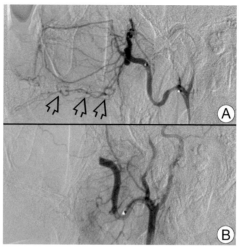

Elderly patient with intractable epistaxis despite nasal packing. A selective distal IMA injection (A) shows atherosclerotic irregularity of distal sphenopalatine branches (arrows), but no active hemorrhage. The vessel was embolized with 250-350 micron PVA and two gelfoam torpedoes (B).

Key Facts
- Procedure definition: Transarterial embolization for intractable nose bleed
  - Anterior epistaxis usually responds to conservative therapy
  - Posterior epistaxis less responsive to conservative therapy & often requires embolization
- Clinical setting triggering procedure
  - Persistent posterior epistaxis despite conservative treatment with nasal packing
    - Usually idiopathic & seen in elderly population
  - Epistaxis with underlying tumor/vascular malformation
    - Hereditary hemorrhagic telangiectasia (HHT)
    - Juvenile nasopharyngeal angiofibroma (JNA)
    - Nasopharyngeal carcinoma
  - Epistaxis 2° to trauma/iatrogenic
    - Post transsphenoidal pituitary resection (usually ICA & life-threatening: May require ICA sacrifice)
- Best procedure approach: Microcatheter embolization of pterygopalatine segment of the internal maxillary artery (IMA) with polyvinyl alcohol (PVA) particles
- Most feared complication(s): CVA/blindness 2° to communication of ECA with ICA or ophthalmic
- Expected outcome: No recurrent epistaxis after unpacking nasal passages in 87-97% of cases

Pre-Procedure
Indications
- Intractable posterior epistaxis

Epistaxis Embolization

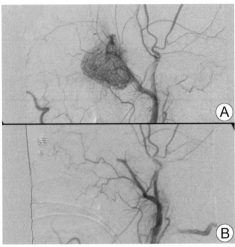

Adolescent male presenting with nasal congestion and epistaxis. An external carotid angiogram (A) shows a hypervascular mass supplied by the distal IMA consistent with a juvenile nasopharyngeal angiofibroma. The tumor was preoperatively embolized with 150-250 micron PVA (B).

<u>Contraindications</u>
- None (only relative contraindications exist in face of life-threatening epistaxis)

<u>Getting Started</u>
- Things to Check
  - CBC, BUN, creatinine, PT, PTT, INR
  - Assess patient's ability to maintain airway & if threatened by ongoing epistaxis, perform embolization under general anesthesia
- Equipment List
  - 6 Fr femoral sheath
  - Standard 5 Fr neuroangiocatheter (Davis, Berenstein, Kerber)
  - 5 or 6 Fr guide catheter
    - Angled tip (Guider, Envoy)
  - Microcatheter/wire
    - Large lumen microcatheter (Renegade, Prowler Plus)
  - Heparinized saline drip (pressurized) for sheath & guide catheter
    - 3,000 IU/liter
  - Rotating hemostatic valve for guide catheter
  - Gelfoam & PVA 150 micron & larger available
    - 1 cc syringes for PVA & Gelfoam

Procedure

<u>Patient Position/Location</u>
- Angio suite with patient supine

<u>Equipment Preparation</u>
- Flush all catheters/sheaths
- Activate hydrophilic coating on catheters/wires by immersion in saline

<u>Procedure Steps</u>
- Access femoral artery & attach flush

Epistaxis Embolization

- Perform common carotid angiogram with neuroangiocatheter to evaluate bifurcation
  - ICA stenosis makes ECA-ICA communication more likely
- Perform ICA angiogram
  - Absence of ophthalmic artery suggests supply from ECA
- Perform ECA angiogram
  - Evaluate for bleeding source (usually none seen)
  - Evaluate for potential ECA-ICA communications
    - Ophthalmic
    - ICA from vidian &/or artery of foramen rotundum
- Exchange for guide catheter & microcatheter/wire which is selectively placed in distal IMA (perform angiogram)
- Embolize to stasis with 250–350 micron PVA (150 -250 if tumor)
  - Mix PVA with 20 cc 240 mgI/ml nonionic contrast
- Gelfoam torpedoes (1–2) injected with 1 cc syringe & contrast
  - Permanent (coil) embolization prevents future interventions
- Evaluate extent of supply to nasal cavity from facial artery with ECA angiogram & embolize with 500–750 micron PVA if necessary
- ENT unpacks nasal passages & observe 30 min for bleeding
- If bleeding embolize opposite IMA/facial with 500 -750 micron PVA
- Standard post angio puncture hemostasis & to PACU for observation

Alternative Procedures/Therapies
- Surgical: Ligation of IMA & ethmoidal arteries

Post-Procedure

Things to Do
- To PACU & admitted minimum 24 hrs
- IV normal saline 75–125 cc/hr until patient is taking adequate p.o. fluids

Things to Avoid
- Excessive activity for first 24 hrs
- Lifting > 50 lbs first 48 hrs
- Immersion of puncture site in water x 5 days

Common Problems & Complications

Problems
- ECA-ICA communications
  - Place microcatheter beyond vessel or protectively embolize communicating vessel with coil(s)
- Ethmoidal (ophthalmic) supply – not accessible for embolization

Complications
- Severe
  - Stroke: Heparinize patient – thrombolysis not effective
  - Septal/skin ischemia: Consider nitroglycerin infusion
- Other complications
  - Cranial neuropathy: Steroid therapy

Selected References
1. Koh E et al: Epistaxis: Vascular anatomy, origins, and endovascular treatment. AJR 174:845-51, 2000
2. Vitek JJ: Idiopathic intractable epistaxis: endovascular therapy. Radiology 181:113-6, 1991
3. Sokoloff J et al: Therapeutic percutaneous embolization in intractable epistaxis. Radiology 111:285-7, 1974

Meningioma Embolization

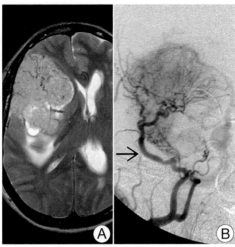

Axial T2 FSE image (A) showing a large pterional meningioma with multiple vascular flow voids, mass effect, edema, and midline shift. Right external carotid angiogram (B) showing an enlarged middle meningeal artery (arrow) as the dominant supply to the tumor.

Key Facts
- Procedure definition: Preoperative embolization of arterial supply to reduce intraoperative blood loss during surgical resection of meningioma
- Clinical setting triggering procedure: Hyper-vascular meningioma
- Best procedure approach: Embolization of meningeal blood supply
- Most feared complication(s): Embolization of non-target areas resulting in stroke or cranial nerve palsies
- Expected outcome
  - Control surgically inaccessible arterial feeders
  - Decrease surgical morbidity by reduction of blood loss & better visualization of surgical field
  - Shorten operative procedure time
  - Increase chance of complete surgical resection
  - Decrease tumor recurrence

Pre-Procedure
<u>Indications</u>
- Meningioma in a location suitable for devascularization
- Palliative temporary necrosis of tumor in inoperable cases

<u>Contraindications</u>
- Absolute contraindications
  - Unsuitable anatomy of arterial supply to tumor
- Relative contraindications
  - Contrast allergy (premedicate)
  - Renal failure
  - Uncorrected coagulopathy

<u>Getting Started</u>
- Things to Check
  - All available neuro-imaging studies: Prior angiograms, MRI, & CT

Meningioma Embolization

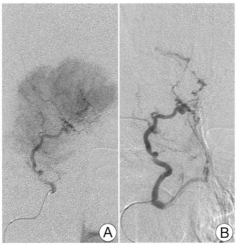

Selective microcatheter injection (A) in the middle meningeal artery prior to embolization. Post embolization run (B) showing marked reduction of arterial supply to the tumor.

- o CBC with platelets, serum electrolytes, BUN, creatinine, PT, PTT, INR
- o If patient has seizures or imaging findings consistent with significant edema consider preoperative steroids &/or anticonvulsant therapy
- o Consider Foley catheter
- Equipment List
  - o 6 Fr arterial sheath
  - o 5 Fr diagnostic neuroangiocatheter
  - o Angled-tip guidewire (0.035" Glidewire)
  - o 5 or 6 Fr guiding catheter (Envoy or Guider)
  - o Large lumen microcatheter (Prowler Plus or Renegade)
  - o Rotating hemostatic valve (RHV) for guide catheter
  - o Microwire (0.014" Transend)
  - o Polyvinyl Alcohol (PVA) particles 45-150 microns & 355-500 microns
  - o Low resistance 1 cc syringes (Medallion) for PVA
  - o Three-way stopcock
  - o 30 cc syringe

Procedure
Patient Position/Location
- Angio suite with patient supine

Equipment Preparation
- Prepare 2 pressurized heparinized saline flush systems (300 mm Hg)
- Flush all sheaths & catheters with heparinized saline

Procedure Steps
- Anesthetize groin and access femoral artery with Seldinger technique
- Place 6 Fr sheath and connect to pressurized drip
- Perform diagnostic angiogram with 5 Fr neuroangiocatheter
  - o Absence of ophthalmic on ICA injection suggests ECA origin
  - o Bilateral ECA injections to evaluate collaterals & vascular supply
- Obtain roadmap & catheterize ECA with guide catheter

Meningioma Embolization

- Attach guide to pressurized heparinized saline using RHV
- Selectively catheterize feeding vessel with microcatheter & microwire
- If catheterizing the middle meningeal artery (MMA), place microcatheter at least 1 cm past the foramen spinosum
  - Reflux of PVA particles < 100 microns in size to foramen spinosum may occlude the petrosal branch of MMA & result in CN VII palsy
- Work in the lateral view for embolization
- Mix PVA: 1 vial to 20 cc of 240 mgI/ml contrast in a 30 cc syringe
- Connect the 30 cc syringe & a 1 cc syringe to a three-way stopcock
- Carefully connect this system to the microcatheter avoiding air bubbles
- Fill the 1 cc syringe from the reservoir of the 30 cc syringe through the three-way stopcock maintaining a closed system
  - The 1 cc syringe can be refilled repeatedly until adequate embolization is achieved
  - Maintain horizontal orientation of syringe barrel to prevent particles from drifting to one end of syringe
- Inject diluted PVA particles (45-150 microns) through microcatheter using 1 cc syringe in short bursts of about 0.3 - 0.4 cc
- Use fluoro to ensure adequate embolization & lack of reflux
- Initial small particles result in central tumor necrosis
- Inject larger PVA particles (355-500 microns)
- Do not use coils if future access should it be necessary (potential subtotal resection)
- Continue injecting until 90% stasis is achieved with some reflux along microcatheter (with care taken not to reflux into non-targeted vessels)
- Clear microcatheter using saline & 1 cc syringe to avoid further reflux

Post-Procedure
Things to Do
- To PACU & admitted minimum 24 hrs
- IV normal saline 75-125 cc/hr until patient is taking adequate p.o. fluids
Things to Avoid
- Excessive activity for first 24 hrs
- Lifting >50 lbs first 48 hrs
- Immersion of puncture site in water x 5 days

Common Problems & Complications
- Catheter or wire induced vasospasm
  - Transdermal nitroglycerine (NTG) paste may prevent spasm
  - Consider IA NTG in 100-200 µg boluses or IA Papaverine 30-60 mg
- Potential collaterals resulting in non-target embolization
- Reflux of particles into non-targeted vessels

Selected References
1. Dean BL et al: Efficacy of endovascular treatment of meningiomas: evaluation with matched samples. AJNR 15: 1675-80, 1994
2. Nelson PK et al: Current status of interventional neuroradiology in the management of meningiomas. Neurosurgery Clin 5: 331-48, 1994
3. Manelfe C et al: Preoperative embolization of intracranial meningiomas. AJNR 5: 963-72, 1986

Paraganglioma Embolization

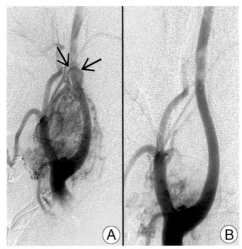

Carotid body tumor. Lateral pre (A) and post (B) embolization angiograms. There is prominent supply to the tumor from the ascending pharyngeal artery (arrows). Several feeders arising from this vessel were embolized. The post embolization angiogram shows residual supply from multiple minute (inaccessible) feeders.

Key Facts
- Procedure definition: Preoperative arterial embolization to reduce blood loss during resection of paraganglioma
- Clinical setting triggering procedure: Paraganglioma
- Best procedure approach: Embolization of ECA blood supply
- Most feared complication(s)
  - Embolization of non-target areas resulting in stroke or cranial nerve palsies
  - Hypertensive crisis
- Expected outcome
  - Control surgically inaccessible arterial feeders
  - Decrease surgical morbidity by reduction of blood loss
  - Shorten operative procedure time
  - Increase chance of complete surgical resection

Pre-Procedure

Indication
- Glomus tympanicum, jugulare, vagale or caroticum

Contraindications
- Absolute contraindication
  - Arterial supply to tumor unsafe for embolization
- Relative contraindications
  - Contrast allergy (premedicate)
  - Renal failure
  - Uncorrected coagulopathy

Getting Started
- Things to Check
  - All available neuro imaging studies: Prior angiograms, MRI, & CT
  - BUN, creatinine, PT, PTT, INR
  - Consider Foley catheter

Paraganglioma Embolization

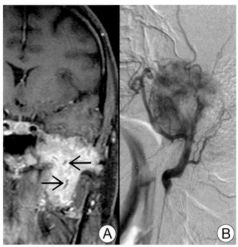

Glomus jugulare. Coronal enhanced T1 image (A) and lateral angiogram (B) showing a hypervascular destructive temporal bone mass with flow voids (arrows) and mass effect upon the temporal lobe. The tumor was embolized with a combination of 150-250 micron PVA particles and Gelfoam.

- Equipment List
  - 6 Fr arterial sheath
  - 5 Fr diagnostic neuroangiocatheter
  - Angled-tip guidewire (0.035" Glidewire)
  - 5 or 6 Fr guiding catheter (Envoy or Guider)
  - Large lumen microcatheter (Prowler Plus or Renegade)
  - Rotating hemostatic valve (RHV) for guide catheter
  - Microwire (0.014" Transend, or Agility)
  - Polyvinyl Alcohol (PVA) particles 150-250 microns & larger depending on degree of arterio-venous shunting through tumor
  - Low resistance 1 cc syringes (Medallion) for PVA
  - Three-way stopcock
  - 30 cc syringe
  - Regitine (phentolamine) available for hypertensive crisis

Procedure

Patient Position/Location
- Angio suite with patient supine

Equipment Preparation
- Prepare 2 pressurized heparinized saline flush systems (300 mm Hg)
- Flush all sheaths & catheters with heparinized saline

Procedure Steps
- Anesthetize groin and access femoral artery with Seldinger technique
- Place 6 Fr sheath and connect to pressurized drip
- Perform diagnostic angiogram with 5 Fr neuroangiocatheter
  - Bilateral ECA injections to evaluate collaterals & vascular supply
  - Ipsilateral vertebral angiography for possible supply to tumor
- Obtain roadmap & catheterize ECA with guide catheter
- Attach guide to pressurized heparinized saline using RHV

Paraganglioma Embolization

- Selectively catheterize feeding vessel with microcatheter & microwire
  - The ascending pharyngeal is often the main feeding vessel & in carotid body tumors drapes over the top of the tumor ("drooping lily")
- Obtain a microcatheter run to look for dangerous collaterals
- If there is a question of cranial nerve injury from embolization a provocative test with lidocaine should be performed
  - Perform baseline cranial nerve exam & inject 20 mg lidocaine into microcatheter & repeat cranial nerve exam
  - If lidocaine causes deficit consider larger particles &/or protective embolization of distal vessel with coils or Gelfoam
- Lateral view often best for embolization
- Mix PVA: 1 vial to 20 cc of 240 mgI/ml contrast in a 30 cc syringe
- Connect the 30 cc syringe & a 1 cc syringe to a three-way stopcock
- Fill the 1 cc syringe from the reservoir of the 30 cc syringe through the three-way stopcock maintaining a closed system
  - The 1 cc syringe can be refilled repeatedly until adequate embolization is achieved
- Inject diluted PVA particles (150-250 microns) through microcatheter using 1 cc syringe in short bursts of about 0.3 - 0.4 cc
- Quickly move to larger particles to close larger feeders/shunts
- Clear microcatheter using saline & 1 cc syringe to avoid reflux
- Coils may be used to occlude large feeders at end of embolization
  - Use Gelfoam pledgets if there is a possibility of only partial resection & need for future embolization (e.g. skull base tumors)

Post-Procedure
Things to Do
- To PACU & admitted minimum 24 hrs
- IV normal saline 75-125 cc/hr until patient is taking adequate p.o. fluids
Things to Avoid
- Excessive activity for first 24 hrs
- Lifting > 50 lbs first 48 hrs
- Immersion of puncture site in water x 5 days

Common Problems & Complications
- Catheter or wire-induced vasospasm
  - Transdermal nitroglycerine (NTG) paste may prevent spasm
  - Consider IA NTG in 100-200 µg boluses or IA Papaverine 30-60 mg
- Potential collaterals resulting in non-target embolization
- Reflux of particles into non-targeted vessels
- Hypertension due to catecholamine release by tumor
  - Phentolamine 2-5 mg IV & additional 1 mg as needed

Selected References
1. Valavanis A: Preoperative embolization of the head and neck: Indications, patient selection, goals, and precautions. AJNR 7: 943-52, 1986
2. Horton JA et al: Lidocaine injection into external carotid branches: Provocative test to preserve cranial nerve function in therapeutic embolization. AJNR 7: 105-8, 1986
3. Hesselink JR et al: Selective arteriography of glomus tympanicum and jugulare tumors: Techniques, normal and pathologic arterial anatomy. AJNR 2: 289-97, 1981

Microcatheter Use

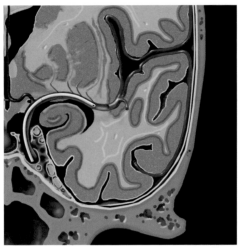

A microcatheter has been advanced to the level of the clot prior to thrombolysis of this middle cerebral artery embolus.

Key Facts
- Clinical setting triggering procedure: Super-selective catheterization for stroke thrombolysis and AVM, aneurysm or tumor embolization
- Best procedure approach: Trans-femoral guiding catheter placement with coaxial super-selective microcatheterization
- Most feared complications
  - Embolic stroke
  - Vessel/aneurysm rupture
  - Microcatheter rupture & unintended embolization of embolic material
- Expected outcome
  - Navigation of tortuous anatomy with desired placement of microcatheter at target level

Pre-Procedure
Indications
- Super-selective catheterization for
  - Aneurysm coiling
  - AVM embolization & super-selective Wada testing
  - Tumor embolization
  - Stroke thrombolysis

Contraindications
- Unsuitable vessel size & overly tortuous anatomy
- Uncorrected coagulopathy
- Renal failure

Getting Started
- Things to Check
  - Imaging studies (CT, MR, & prior angio)
  - BUN, creatinine, PT, PTT, INR
- Equipment List
  - Angiography suite
  - 6 Fr sheath

Microcatheter Use

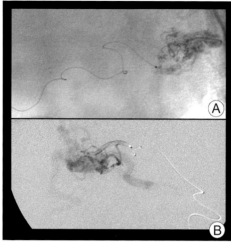

Examples of flow directed and over the wire micro-catheterization. A flow directed microcatheter (A) was used to gain distal access and perform an intra-nidal injection of n-BCA in this AVM supplied by the PCA. An over the wire microcatheter (B) was used to select a specific MCA pedicle supplying this AVM.

- 5 or 6 Fr guiding catheter (Guider, Target; Envoy, Cordis; Northstar, Cook)
- 0.035" angled tip glidewire
- 2 rotating hemostatic valves (RHV)
- 3 heparinized saline pressure bags (inflated to 300 mm Hg)
- Plastic IV cannula (18-20 gauge) attached to flush syringe for irrigation of microcatheter hub
- Microcatheter (2 basic types): Over the wire (OTW) & flow directed
  - OTW microcatheter: 2-3 Fr with inner diameter of 0.010" to 0.027" (Excelsior & Renegade, Target; Prowler, Cordis)
  - OTW microcatheters used for precise placement in a specific location (e.g. aneurysm, clot, vascular supply to tumor)
  - Flow directed: 1.5-1.8 Fr with inner diameter of approx 0.010" (Ultraflow, MTI; Regatta, Cordis; Elite, Target)
  - Flow directed used for distal placement (e.g. for liquid/particle AVM embolization) & carried there by high flow
- Microwire: 0.008"–0.010" for flow directed & 0.010"–0.014" for OTW

Procedure
Equipment Preparation
- Flush all catheters/sheaths
- Activate hydrophilic coating on catheters/wires by immersion in saline
  - Flush plastic container holding microcatheter before removal

Procedure Steps
- Access femoral artery & place femoral sheath & attach flush
- Guide is placed in proximal supplying vessel & flush attached
- Control angiogram obtained
  - Steam shaping of OTW microcatheter performed to facilitate catheterization (Prowler available in various angled tips)

Microcatheter Use

- Shaping mandrel inserted in tip & shaped & placed under steam for < 30 sec (tip is then rapidly dipped in flush bowl to fix shape)
  - o For flow directed a microwire is inserted to tip for support
- Microcatheter & wire (with RHV & flush attached) inserted under roadmapping
  - o For OTW system the wire precedes the catheter by several cm & once wire is in desired location microcatheter is advanced
  - o For flow directed system wire tip is withdrawn to stiff segment of catheter and tip is allowed to be carried distally
- Plastic IV cannula with flush syringe attached is used to irrigate microcatheter hub during wire removal & clear air bubbles/blood

Post-Procedure
Things to Do
- Routine post-angiography orders

Common Problems & Complications
Problems
- Unable to advance OTW catheter through tortuous anatomy
  - o Gentle to & fro motion of wire facilitates microcatheter advancement
  - o Care must be taken if advancement of catheter at groin is unaccompanied by advancement at tip since energy may build in the system & result in sudden & uncontrolled distal movement of tip – remove all slack from system so this does not occur
- Unable to advance flow-directed catheter through tortuous anatomy
  - o Appropriate diameter microwire may be advanced beyond tip as in an OTW system
  - o Small bursts of contrast through a 1 cc syringe will usually redirect tip distally
- Unable to withdraw microcatheter due to spasm/tortuosity (rare)
  - o Heparinize & with continued gentle traction & altered guide wire position catheter should release
  - o Consider nitropaste/nifedipine
  - o Consider papaverine/nitroglycerine infusion
Complications
- Embolic stroke
- Vessel/aneurysm rupture
- Microcatheter rupture & unintended embolization of embolic material

Selected References
1. Zoarski GH et al: Performance Characteristics of microcatheter systems in a standardized tortuous pathway. AJNR 19:1571-6, 1998
2. Aletich VA et al: Arteriovenous malformation nidus catheterization with hydrophilic wire and flow directed catheter. AJNR 18: 929-35, 1997
3. Mathis JM et al: Hydrophilic coatings diminish adhesion of glue to catheter: An in vitro simulation of NBCA embolization. AJNR 18:1087-91, 1997

Papaverine for Vasospasm

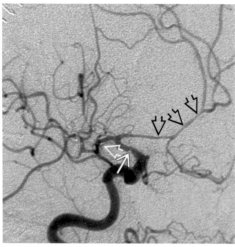

Right carotid injection in a patient with history of SAH from right MCA aneurysm (clipped). Patient developed left-sided weakness, altered mental status & elevated TCD velocities nine days after presentation. There is significant vasospasm of ICA (white arrow), ACA (black open arrows), and MCA (white open arrow).

Key Facts
- Procedure definition: Intra-arterial papaverine (a benzylisoquinoline alkaloid vasodilator) for vasospasm
  - Vasospasm is leading cause of disability & death after intracranial aneurysm rupture
- Clinical setting triggering procedure: Symptomatic vasospasm (progressive neurologic deficits) 2° to subarachnoid hemorrhage
  - Vasospasm usually begins on day 3, maximal at 6-8 days & resolves around 12th day following SAH
- Best procedure approach: Infusion of distal ICA or vertebral artery (VA)
- Most feared complication(s): Embolic complications (crystal formation) & reperfusion hemorrhage of infarcted areas (rare)
- Expected outcome: Restoration of vessel diameter & blood flow (often transient requiring treatment on consecutive days)

Pre-Procedure
Indications
- Symptomatic vasospasm 2° to subarachnoid hemorrhage
  - Refractory to medical therapy
    - Triple H therapy: Hemodilution, hypertension, & hypervolemia
    - Calcium antagonists: Nimodipine (60 mg q 4 hrs x 21 days)
  - As adjunct to angioplasty (which has more durable results)
    - Distal vessels (not amenable to angioplasty): Beyond A1, M2 & P1
    - Facilitate balloon access (proximal vessels with severe vasospasm)
    - Papaverine infusion alone resulted in clinical improvement in only 25% of patients in some studies
Contraindications
- Large region(s) of infarction/hemorrhage
- Refractory hypotension

Papaverine for Vasospasm

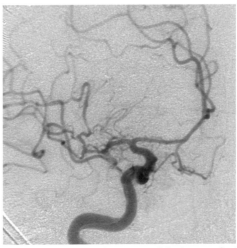

Note is made of marked improvement in vasospasm following supraclinoid infusion of 180 mg of papaverine.

Getting Started
- Things to Check
  - o Patient's neurologic status to predict involved vascular territories
  - o Transcranial Doppler (TCD) velocities
    - A sudden increase in TCD > 120 cm/sec or MCA/ICA ratio of > 3 correlate with onset of vasospasm (> 6 = severe spasm)
  - o CT for infarction, hemorrhage or hydrocephalus
  - o Availability of anesthesia if patient unable to cooperate
  - o BUN, creatinine, PT, PTT, INR
  - o Baseline intracranial pressure (ICP) if possible
- Equipment List
  - o Angiography suite
  - o Ability to monitor ICP if patient has ventriculostomy
  - o 5 French neuroangiography catheter & 0.035" angled tip glidewire
  - o 6 French guiding catheter
  - o 0.018" or 0.021" lumen microcatheter & microwire

Procedure
Procedure Steps
- Access femoral artery & perform diagnostic angiogram
  - o Assess presence & extent of vasospasm
    - Proximal & accessible vessels usually treated with angioplasty
- Treat symptomatic side first by accessing external carotid with exchange glidewire & advancing guiding catheter into common carotid, then select ICA & place guide catheter in distal cervical ICA
  - o ICA is prone to spasm in these patients & hyperdynamic state (guide catheter motion) can predispose to dissection
- Use an oblique magnified roadmap to place microwire/catheter in supraclinoid ICA
  - o Place microcatheter above ophthalmic artery to avoid eye complications & inject microcatheter with contrast to assess where papaverine will go

Papaverine for Vasospasm

- ▪ Sub-selective catheterization may be performed (A1, M1, or P1)
- Mix & infuse papaverine
  - ○ 300 mg/100 cc NS @ 3 cc/min X 30 min = 270 mg
    - ▪ In-line mannitol filter may be used to reduce injection of crystals
    - ▪ Maximum of 300 mg per vascular territory (or 600 mg total dose)
    - ▪ Frequent checks to ensure catheter has not pulled back to ophthalmic artery
    - ▪ Check progress via guide catheter injections q 5-10 min (endpoint is restored vessel diameter, normal transit time or 300 mg/vessel)
- Alternative method
  - ○ 600 mg/500 cc NS & infuse by intermittent 3 cc boluses q 20 seconds
    - ▪ This decreases laminar flow & should improve distribution of drug

Alternative Procedures/Therapies
- Radiologic
  - ○ Balloon angioplasty more effective & usually performed for proximal vessel vasospasm (combination of two therapies frequently used)

Post-Procedure
Things to Do
- Femoral arterial sheath generally left in place (attached to a normal saline flush) for repeat treatments on subsequent days
- Patient is returned to neuro intensive care & frequent neuro checks are performed

Common Problems & Complications
Problems
- Monitor for hypotension/tachycardia & adjust infusion
- Monitor ICP & adjust infusion
  - ○ Maintain cerebral perfusion pressure (mean arterial pressure – ICP) ≥ 60 mm Hg as ICP rises by slowing infusion
- Effects may be short lived compared with angioplasty & may require daily infusions

Complications
- Severe
  - ○ Reperfusion hemorrhage
  - ○ Blindness from retinal artery occlusion
  - ○ Transient neurologic dysfunction
  - ○ Papaverine precipitation & emboli
  - ○ Paradoxical worsening of vasospasm
  - ○ Severe brainstem function depression (with VA infusions)
- Other complications
  - ○ Elevated ICP (adjust infusion rate downward)
  - ○ Hypotension & tachycardia
  - ○ Mydriasis

Selected References
1. Cross DT III et al: Intracranial pressure monitoring during intraarterial papaverine infusion for cerebral vasospasm. AJNR 19:1319-23, 1998
2. Eskridge JM: A practical approach to the treatment of vasospasm. AJNR 18:1653-60, 1997
3. Clouston JE et al: Intraarterial papaverine infusion for cerebral vasospasm after subarachnoid hemorrhage. AJNR 16:27-38, 1995

Spinal Angiogram

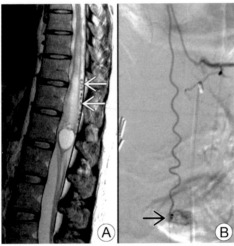

Von Hippel-Lindau syndrome. Sagittal thoraco-lumbar T2 FSE (A) showing a cystic mass, cord expansion, and edema with enlarged draining veins dorsally (arrows). AP angiogram (B) showing an enlarged artery of Adamkiewicz supplying the tumor nodule (black arrow). Hemangioblastoma was found at surgery.

Key Facts
- Clinical setting triggering procedure: Suspected vascular pathology of the spine and/or spinal cord
- Best procedure approach: Trans-femoral catheterization of arterial supply to spine & spinal cord
- Most feared complication: Cord infarction
- Expected outcome: Diagnosis & treatment of vascular abnormalities involving the spinal axis

Pre-Procedure
Indications
- Suspected vascular malformation
  - Spinal dural arteriovenous fistula (SDAVF) most common
    - Patients present with MR/clinical symptoms of venous congestion of the cord
  - Intramedullary spinal AVM
  - Perimedullary arteriovenous fistula
- SAH with negative cerebral angiography x 2
- Preoperative/palliative embolization of hypervascular vertebral body tumor
- Mapping of spinal arteries prior to spine surgery
Contraindications
- Uncorrected coagulopathy
- Renal failure
Getting Started
- Things to Check
  - Imaging studies (MR, & prior angio)
  - BUN, creatinine, PT, PTT, INR
- Equipment List
  - Angiography suite

Spinal Angiogram

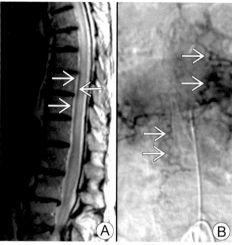

Spinal dural arteriovenous fistula (SDAVF). Sagittal thoraco-lumbar T2 FSE (A) showing cord edema and peripheral hypointensity (arrows) secondary to venous congestion. AP angiogram (B) showing enlarged early draining veins (arrows). The patient was treated with combined embolization (PVA) and surgery.

- o 5 Fr sheath
- o 5 Fr spinal angiocatheter
    - ▪ HS-1 or HS-2
    - ▪ H1H Headhunter
    - ▪ Mikaelsson
- o 0.035" angled tip glidewire

Procedure

Patient Position/Location
- Angio suite with patient supine

Equipment Preparation
- Flush all catheters/sheaths
- Activate hydrophilic coating on catheters/wires by immersion in saline

Procedure Steps
- A long ruler with radiopaque numbers is placed from upper thoracic spine to S1 & contiguous preliminary images are recorded
- Access femoral artery & place femoral sheath
- If a specific level is to be studied (e.g. spine metastasis embolization) that level & 2 levels above & below are studied for tumor & spinal cord arterial supply
- If the entire spinal axis is to be studied (e.g. SDAVF or AVM) then each intercostal & lumbar is studied
    - o An assistant records each injection on the preliminary images to assure all vessels are studied
    - o Complete study of vascular supply to the cord also includes evaluation of vertebral, common carotid, subclavian (thyrocervical & costocervical), & median sacral arteries
    - o Artery of Adamkiewicz usually arises from a left intercostal artery between T9 & L2

Spinal Angiogram

- A contrast syringe is attached to the spinal angiocatheter and the origins of the intercostal/lumbar arteries are sought
  - The vessels usually originate posterolaterally just below pedicles & are upwardly directed in the upper spine & downwardly directed in the lower spine
  - The origins are increasingly posterior in the lower spine & may have a common trunk in the lumbar spine
- Tip of catheter will fall into origin & confirmation with gentle injection of contrast is made & catheter is then seated by withdrawing slightly
- Hand injection run is performed with 0.5–2 cc of nonionic contrast
- Procedure is repeated until all vessels are studied or contrast limit is reached
- Standard post-angiogram orders & patient transferred to recovery

Alternative Procedures/Therapies
- Radiologic: MRI

Post-Procedure
Things to Do
- Patients usually observed in PACU 6–8 hrs & discharged if stable
- IV normal saline 75–125 cc/hr until patient is taking adequate p.o. fluids

Things to Avoid
- Excessive activity for first 24 hrs
- Lifting > 50 lbs first 48 hrs
- Immersion of puncture site in water x 5 days

Common Problems & Complications
Problems
- Contrast limits may require 2 sessions
- Difficulty with catheterization
  - Both intercostal/lumbar arteries at a single level may originate from the right or left of the aorta due to ectasia/tortuosity
  - Aorta tapers caudally & upper arteries are directed cephalad & lower arteries caudad which may require 2 different catheters (i.e. H1H for upper thoracic & HS-1 for lumbar)

Complications
- Cord infarction

Selected References
1. Berkefeld J et al: Hypervascular spinal tumors: Influence of the embolization technique on perioperative hemorrhage. AJNR 20:757-63, 1999
2. Champlin AM et al: Preoperative spinal angiography for lateral extracavitary approach to thoracic and lumbar spine. AJNR 15:73-7, 1994
3. Enzmann DR et al: Intraarterial digital subtraction spinal angiography. AJNR 4:25-6, 1983

Stroke Thrombolysis

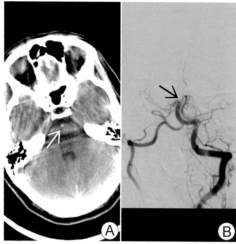

Acute vertebrobasilar thromboembolic stroke. CT without contrast (A) showing a dense basilar artery sign (arrow). Left vertebral arteriogram (B) showing thrombus in the distal basilar artery (black arrow).

Key Facts
- Procedure definition: Thrombolysis in setting of acute ischemic stroke
- Stroke is third most frequent cause of death & leading cause of disability
- IV and intra-arterial (IA) routes of thrombolytic agents are used clinically
- Most feared complication: Hemorrhagic transformation (HT)
- Expected outcome: 66% MCA recanalization rate in PROACT II trial

Pre-Procedure
Indications for IA Therapy
- Acute ischemic stroke during angiography
- Acute ischemic stroke presenting beyond 3 hr time window for IV therapy
  - CTA & perfusion CT can expedite treatment by characterizing level of arterial occlusion & defining ischemic tissue at risk of infarction
    - Proximal MCA (M1) thrombus is less responsive to IV therapy
  - MRI demonstrating diffusion-perfusion mismatch (tissue at risk) useful but often not time effective
  - In general time of onset of symptoms to completion of IA therapy should not exceed 6-9 hrs for anterior circulation
  - Window for vertebrobasilar circulation IA thrombolysis may be extended to 24-48 hrs or longer depending on clinical setting

Contraindications
- Intracranial hemorrhage (absolute)
- CT evidence of completed infarction involving ≥ 1/3 of vascular territory correlates with increased risk of HT
  - Mechanical clot disruption or extraction may be considered
- Recent surgery or trauma (relative)
- Pregnancy (relative)

Getting Started
- Obtain informed consent & counsel family on risks/benefits of procedure
- Consult with stroke neurologist

Stroke Thrombolysis

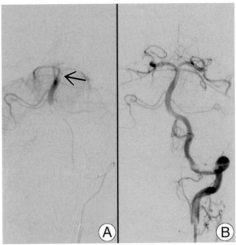

(A) Partial lysis of clot in the basilar artery revealing focal residual thrombus (arrow). (B) Further thrombolysis showing a completely recanalized basilar artery. The patient made a full recovery (case courtesy Richard Wiggins, MD).

- Things to Check
  - CT for evidence of hemorrhage/low density
  - Baseline CBC, PT, PTT, INR, BUN, creatinine
- Equipment List
  - Angiography suite
  - 5 French neuroangiography catheter & 0.035" angled-tip glidewire
  - 6 French guiding catheter & microcatheter/microwire
  - At least 0.018" lumen microcatheter preferred allowing microsnare use
  - Compliant angioplasty balloon, microsnare (retrieval device)
- Medications
  - Alteplase (rt-PA)
    - Total IA dose ≤ 20 mg (& often ≤ 10 mg) may be effective
    - Avoid mixing with heparin or contrast
    - Dilution beyond 0.2 mg/ml not recommended by manufacturer
  - Reteplase (r-PA)
    - 1 unit initial dose then 0.1-1 unit/hr
    - Longer half-life life than rt-PA
    - Greater clot penetration than rt-PA due to less fibrin affinity
    - May dilute 10 U in 100 ml of NS (0.1 U/ml)
  - GP IIb/IIIa inhibitors
    - Particularly useful for thrombo-emboli during stenting/coiling
    - May facilitate recanalization when used with rt-PA or r-PA
    - Abciximab dose: 0.25 mg/kg initial IV bolus without 12 hr infusion (low dose IA has been used in 5-10 mg range)
    - Avoid concomitant heparin use
  - Heparin
    - Low dose (if used): 2,000 IU IV bolus & 500 IU/hr IV

Stroke Thrombolysis

Procedure
Patient Preparation
- Ensure patient is stable & consult anesthesia if unable to maintain airway
  - Oxygen @ 12 L/min by facemask; IV normal saline

Procedure Steps
- Access femoral artery & perform 3 vessel angiogram
  - Assess presence & level of occlusion
  - Assess extent of collaterals
  - Finish angiogram with catheter in vessel supplying affected territory
- Exchange for guiding catheter attached to heparinized saline flush
- Advance microcatheter & wire beyond occlusion (if possible)
  - Consider snare retrieval of clot
  - 1/3 of initial thrombolytic dose administered distal, 1/3 laced into clot, & 1/3 proximal to clot
  - Several passes of microcatheter/wire will help recanalization
- Frequent angiographic runs to check progress & need for additional agent(s)
- End point: Recanalization or time/dose limits

Post-Procedure
Things to Do
- Admit to ICU
- CBC 2-4 hrs & 24 hrs following procedure to exclude thrombocytopenia 2° to heparin or IIb/IIIa inhibitor effects
- CT to assess for HT (contrast staining of ischemic territory frequent & should not be confused with HT)
- Femoral arterial sheath generally left in place 12-24 hrs (pull when ACT ≤ 180) or consider a closure device

Common Problems & Complications
Problems
- Clot resistant to lysis
  - Consider adding IIb/IIIa inhibitor &/or macerating clot with wire, balloon, or snare

Complications
- Hemorrhagic transformation risk increases with
  - Time to treatment
  - Low density/mass effect on CT involving ≥ 1/3 of involved vascular territory
  - Stroke severity based on NIHSS
  - High heparin dose used in combination with thrombolytics
  - Absent collateral perfusion from surrounding vascular territories
  - Low platelet count
  - Glucose ≥ 200

Selected References
1. Kwon O et al: Intraarterially administered abciximab as an adjuvant thrombolytic therapy: Report of three cases. AJNR 23:447-51, 2002
2. Eckert B et al: Acute basilar artery occlusion treated with combined intravenous abciximab and intra-arterial tissue plasminogen Activator. Stroke 33:1424, 2002
3. Zeumer H et al: Local intraarterial thrombolysis in vertebrobasilar thromboembolic disease. AJNR 4:401-4, 1983

Vertebral Angiogram

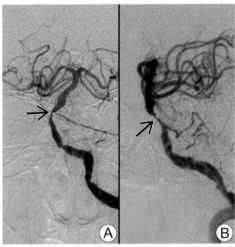

Basilar artery stenosis. AP (A) and lateral (B) left vertebral angiogram in a patient presenting with posterior fossa TIA's. A high grade basilar artery stenosis (arrows) is identified at the origin of the left anterior inferior cerebellar artery. The lesion was treated with angioplasty (not shown).

Key Facts
- Clinical setting triggering procedure: Suspected vascular abnormality involving the vertebrobasilar territory
- Best procedure approach: Transfemoral catheterization of subclavian (SA) & vertebral artery (VA)
- Most feared complications
  - Embolic stroke
  - VA Dissection
- Expected outcome
  - Angiographic evaluation of entire vertebrobasilar circulation (including contralateral distal VA)

Pre-Procedure
Indications
- Vertebrobasilar insufficiency (VBI)
- Subclavian steal
- 4 vessel angiographic workup for SAH
- Post-traumatic dissection
- Pre-operative or pre-embolization workup of cervical, posterior fossa, or supratentorial neoplasm/vascular lesion
- Vasculitis workup
Contraindications
- Uncorrected coagulopathy
- Renal failure
Getting Started
- Things to Check
  - Imaging studies (CT, MR, US, & prior angio)
  - BUN, creatinine, PT, PTT, INR
- Equipment List
  - Angiography suite

Vertebral Angiogram

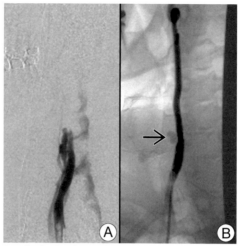

Vertebral artery fistula. A right vertebral artery fistula developed after attempted central line placement. Right vertebral angiogram (A) shows prompt filling of perivertebral and spinal epidural veins. (B) The fistula was successfully closed with a single detachable balloon (arrow).

- o 5 Fr sheath
- o 5 Fr Pigtail catheter
- o 5 Fr neuroangiography catheter with a hockey-stick type tip
  - Berenstein, Davis, or Vert catheters
  - H1H Headhunter useful for right VA
- o 0.035" angled-tip glidewire

Procedure
Patient Position/Location
- Angio suite with patient supine
Equipment Preparation
- Flush all catheters/sheaths
- Activate hydrophilic coating on catheters/wires by immersion in saline
Procedure Steps
- Access femoral artery & place femoral sheath
- An LAO aortic arch angiogram is performed in most instances (SAH, tumor, & vascular malformation workup the exceptions)
  - o VAs are evaluated for stenosis & safety of selective catheterization
- Selective SA injection may be needed to further define VA origin
  - o Slight ipsilateral & caudal angulation helpful for tortuous origins
- Left VA (dominant in 40% of patients) usually selected
  - o Left VA usually arises from superior aspect of SA but may originate from more proximal medial aspect of SA
- Gentle probing of origin with glidewire will usually allow passage of wire to the C4-5 level
  - o Use road mapping if any difficulty is encountered
  - o Full inspiration may facilitate wire passage through tortuous VA
- Selection of right VA may be difficult due to SA tortuosity
  - o Creating a gentle C-curve at wire tip may facilitate SA catheterization

Vertebral Angiogram

- o Once catheter is beyond VA the origin can be sought with gentle contrast injection during pullback of catheter
- Advance catheter to C6 & double flush & check run-off
  - o If tortuous, advancing catheter in concert with cardiac cycle may help
  - o Contrast stasis may be seen due to spasm, tortuosity or stenosis
    - If stasis is encountered pull catheter back while gently injecting contrast until run-off resumes or catheter is out of VA
    - If selective run can not be performed safely switch to contralateral VA or perform run with catheter in subclavian & brachial BP cuff inflated above systolic
- Contrast injection rates vary with VA caliber: 4-6 cc/sec for 5-9 cc
  - o If VA ends in PICA a gentle hand injection is preferable
- Goal is to reflux contralateral VA to level of PICA
  - o Placing catheter in more distal cervical VA increases reflux if necessary
- Perform run in Towne's view for posterior cerebral arteries
  - o AP/slight Water's view best demonstrates basilar artery/posterior fossa
- Standard post-cerebral angiogram orders & patient transferred to recovery

Alternative Procedures/Therapies
- Radiologic
  - o MRA
  - o CTA
  - o Doppler ultrasound for the V1 & V2 segments

Post-Procedure

Things to Do
- Patients usually observed in PACU 6–8 hrs & discharged if stable & ambulating
- IV normal saline 75–125 cc/hr until patient is taking adequate p.o. fluids

Things to Avoid
- Excessive activity for first 24 hrs
- Lifting > 50 lbs first 48 hrs
- Immersion of puncture site in water x 5 days

Common Problems & Complications

Problems
- VA may originate from aorta in 5%
- Tortuous anatomy preventing catheterization
  - o Perform run with catheter in SA & brachial BP cuff inflated above systolic
  - o If selective catheterization is mandatory perform retrograde brachial catheterization

Complications
- Dissection and/or stroke

Selected References
1. Yousem DM et al: Injection rates for neuroangiography: Results of a survey. AJNR 22:1838-40, 2001
2. Osborn AG: Diagnostic cerebral angiography-2nd ed. Philadelphia. Lippincott Williams & Wilkins. 1999
3. Nogueira TE et al: Dual origin of the vertebral artery mimicking dissection. AJNR 18:382-4, 1997

Inferior Petrosal Sinus Sampling

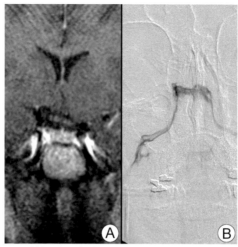

Thirty-eight year-old female with a long history of Cushing syndrome. The stimulation and suppression tests pointed to a pituitary source, but the MRI (A) was equivocal. Right IPS injection (B) shows reflux into the contralateral IPS.

Key Facts
- Procedure definition: Bilateral simultaneous inferior petrosal sinus (IPS) sampling before and after administration of IV ovine corticotropin-releasing hormone (oCRH)
- Clinical setting triggering procedure: To determine pituitary (Cushing disease) vs. ectopic source of ACTH-dependent Cushing syndrome
- Best procedure approach: Bilateral IPS catheter placement by way of both femoral veins
- Most feared complication(s): IPS thrombosis, brainstem injury, subarachnoid hemorrhage
- Expected outcome
  - Differentiation between pituitary (adenoma) & non-pituitary (ectopic) source of ACTH secretion
  - Pre-op lateralization of ACTH secretion from pituitary gland

Pre-Procedure
Indications
- To determine pituitary (Cushing disease) vs ectopic source of ACTH-dependent Cushing syndrome
  - MRI of pituitary equivocal or normal
  - Peripheral ACTH sampling equivocal after oCRH stimulation & dexamethasone suppression tests
- Persistent Cushing syndrome following transsphenoidal surgery
Contraindications
- Uncorrected coagulopathy
- Systemic or local (groin) infection
- Contrast allergy (relative: Premedicate or use gadolinium)
Getting Started
- Things to check
  - BUN, creatinine, PT, PTT, INR

Inferior Petrosal Sinus Sampling

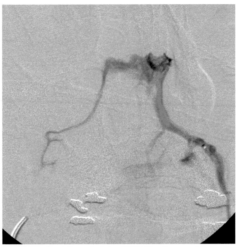

Left IPS injection with reflux into contralateral IPS. Simultaneous bilateral and peripheral ACTH levels were drawn before and after oCRH administration. Lab results showed a ratio of IPS:peripheral ACTH greater than 3, and a right:left IPS ACTH of greater than 1.4.

- o Review prior endocrine workup & relevant lab results
- o Review MR of pituitary
- Equipment List
  - o 6 French femoral sheath
  - o Two angiocatheters
    - ▪ 4 French angled-tip catheters such as Davis or Berenstein
  - o 0.035" angled-tip glidewire
  - o Alternative: Two 5 or 6 Fr guide catheters (Guider, Envoy or Northstar)
    - ▪ Use with large lumen microcatheters (Renegade or Prowler Plus) and a microwire

Procedure
Patient Position/Location
- Angio suite with patient supine

Equipment Preparation
- Flush all catheters/sheaths
- Activate hydrophilic coating on catheters/wires by immersion in saline
- Confirm oCRH (Acthrel) is available

Procedure Steps
- 6 French right femoral sheath placed (micropuncture system for access)
- Angiocatheter placed in left groin
- IV heparin 3,000 to 5,000 IU & 1,000 to 2,000 IU q hr
- Advance left femoral catheter through heart (monitor EKG for arrhythmias) & into left innominate
- Left internal jugular (IJ) selected by probing with glidewire
- Advance catheter to jugular bulb & select IPS which enters anteromedial aspect of IJ just before IJ turns posteriorly
  - o Forceful injection of contrast with catheter in IJ may reflux IPS for road-mapping

Inferior Petrosal Sinus Sampling

- Similar technique used to place catheter in right IPS
  - Injection of left IPS will often reflux down right IPS for localization
- Document proper position of catheters with angiographic runs
- Simultaneous 2 cc samples are drawn from both IPSs and right femoral sheath 5 & 1 min prior to oCRH (1 µg/kg IV) & 2, 5, & 10 min after
  - Waste dead-space volume of catheters/sheath prior to each draw
  - Flush catheters between draws
  - Samples are submitted to lab in lavender-topped vials on ice
- Document catheters are still in each IPS at end of study
- Remove catheters/sheath & apply pressure for hemostasis for 10 – 15 min

Interpreting Results
- Cushing disease (pituitary source): 2:1 IPS:peripheral ACTH ratio pre-oCRH & 3:1 ratio post-oCRH
- Interpetrosal ratio of $\geq$ 1.4 to lateralize

Post-Procedure
Things to Do
- Observe in PACU minimum of 4 hrs
- IV normal saline 75–125 cc/hr until patient is taking adequate p.o. fluids

Things to Avoid
- Excessive activity for first 24 hrs
- Lifting > 50 lbs first 48 hrs
- Immersion of puncture site in water x 5 days

Common Problems & Complications
Problems
- IPS has a variable entrance into IJ
  - Search more inferiorly with catheter (forceful injection with lower catheter position while compressing ipsilateral IJ may show IPS)
- IPS may be hypoplastic or not drain to IJ

Complications
- Severe
  - IPS thrombosis – prophylactic heparinization
  - Injury to brainstem venous drainage from excessive wire/microcatheter probing or overly forceful injection in IPS
  - Wire/catheter perforation & SAH – microcatheter less traumatic & maintain wire/catheter below IPS/cavernous sinus junction
- Other complications
  - Puncture site bleeding – rare if micropuncture system used for access

Selected References
1. Bonelli FS et al: Adrenocorticotropic hormone-dependent Cushing's Syndrome: Sensitivity and Specificity of Inferior Petrosal Sinus Sampling. AJNR 21:690-6, 2000
2. Oliverio PJ et al: Bilateral simultaneous cavernous sinus sampling using corticotropin-releasing hormone in the evaluation of Cushing disease. AJNR 17:1669-74, 1996
3. Oldfield et al: Petrosal sinus sampling with and without corticotropin-releasing hormone for the differential diagnosis of Cushing's Syndrome. NEJM 325:897-905, 1991

Vertebral Stenting

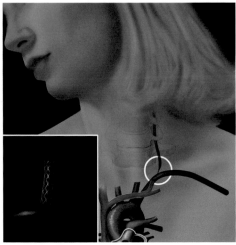

Tight left vertebral artery origin stenosis treated with stenting (inset).

Key Facts
- Procedure definition: Endovascular vertebral artery (VA) revascularization
- Clinical setting triggering procedure
  - Symptomatic VA stenosis > 70% with contralateral VA occlusion or stenosis of equal or greater severity
- Best procedure approach: Transfemoral sheath placed in subclavian with balloon expandable stent placement
- Most feared complications
  - Embolic stroke
  - Rupture of VA
  - Acute stent thrombosis
- Expected outcome
  - < 20% residual stenosis
  - Absence of recurrent neurologic symptoms

Pre-Procedure
Indications
- Symptomatic > 70% VA stenosis with contra-lateral VA occlusion or stenosis of equal or greater severity
  - Patients have generally failed antiplatelet/anticoagulant therapy
  - High incidence of recoil & restenosis with angioplasty alone (particularly with ostial lesions)
- Symptomatic VA dissection
- VA pseudoaneurysm/dissecting aneurysm
Contraindications
- Uncorrected coagulopathy
- Recent infarction
- Angiographic evidence of thrombus at level of stenosis
- Renal failure
Getting Started
- Things to Check
  - Imaging studies (CT, MR, US, & prior angio)

Vertebral Stenting

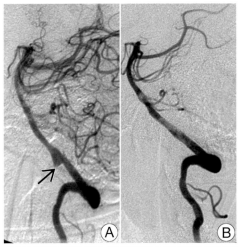

Lateral view left vertebral angiogram (A) showing a dissecting aneurysm of the V4 segment (arrow) in a patient who presented with SAH. After placement of a 3 mm Radius stent the aneurysm no longer fills (B).

-     o BUN, creatinine, PT, PTT, INR
- Medications
  - o Aspirin 325 mg daily commencing 4 days prior to procedure
  - o Clopidogrel (Plavix) 75 mg daily commencing 4 days prior to procedure
  - o Heparin 5,000 IU (maintain ACT twice baseline) prior to placing guide
  - o Hydrate with IV normal saline
- Equipment List
  - o Angiography suite
  - o 7 Fr sheath with pigtail & neuroangiography catheter & 0.035" angled tip glidewire
  - o 7 Fr guiding catheter (Envoy, Cordis Endovascular; Guider, Target)
  - o Microcatheter (Renegade, Target; Rapid Transit, Cordis Endovascular)
  - o 0.014" microwire (Transend, Target)
  - o 0.018" exchange microwire
  - o 2 or 3 mm low profile angioplasty balloon (Savvy; Cordis Endovascular)
  - o 3 to 5 mm balloon expandable stent (Bx Velocity, Cordis Endovascular; NIR, Boston Scientific Target; or S7, AVE Medtronic)
  - o For dissection/dissecting aneurysm a 3 to 5 mm balloon expandable stent may be desirable (Radius, Boston Scientific; or Magic Wallstent, Schneider)

Procedure
Patient Position/Location
- Angio suite with patient supine
- Radiopaque marker is placed on ipsilateral neck for measurements
Equipment Preparation
- Flush all catheters/sheaths
- Activate hydrophilic coating on catheters/wires by immersion in saline

Vertebral Stenting

Procedure Steps
- Foley inserted
- Access femoral artery & perform 4 vessel angiogram
  - Assess collaterals & establish baseline appearance of intracranial vasculature
  - Measure stenosis & select balloon that is 1 mm smaller than normal VA diameter
    - If stenosis is < 80% pre-dilation may not be necessary
- Select subclavian with glidewire & 7 Fr guide catheter
  - Brachial approach may be necessary if tortuous (usually on right)
- A second guide wire may be placed out the subclavian/axillary artery to stabilize guiding catheter if necessary
- Cross stenosis with 0.014" wire & microcatheter & exchange for 0.018" wire
- Pre-dilate if necessary
- Exchange for & deploy stent & perform angiogram with wire across stent
  - Assess need for additional post-stent angioplasty
- Final intracranial angio to exclude embolic complication
- Heparin discontinued & sheath removed when ACT < 180 (or closure device is used)

Alternative Procedures/Therapies
- Surgical: VA reimplantation

Post-Procedure
Things to Do
- Admit to ICU x 24 Hrs with close monitoring of neuro status
- Plavix 75 mg/day x 4–6 weeks & aspirin 325 mg/day indefinitely

Common Problems & Complications
Problems
- Dissection during angioplasty may require placement of additional stents
- Tortuous anatomy may require brachial approach
- High incidence of neo-intimal hyperplasia & restenosis

Complications
- Stroke (distal protection devices currently in trials)
- Rupture of VA
- Acute stent thrombosis
- Stent infection

Selected References
1. Kirsch EC et al: Carotid arterial stent placement: Results and follow-up in 53 Patients. Radiology 220:737-44, 2001
2. Phatouros CC et al: Endovascular stenting for carotid artery stenosis: Preliminary experience using the Shape-Memory-Alloy-Recoverable-Technology (SMART) stent. AJNR 21:732-8, 2000
3. Vitek JJ et al: Carotid artery stenting: Technical considerations. AJNR 21:1736-43, 2000

Wada Test

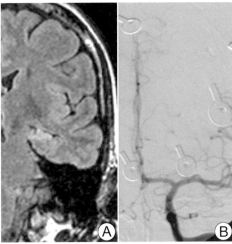

Patient with a longstanding history of partial complex seizure disorder. (A) Coronal FLAIR image shows increased signal in the left hippocampus consistent with mesial temporal sclerosis. (B) AP view of LICA angiogram showing no abnormal vascular contribution to basilar artery and no significant cross-filling of opposite ACA.

Key Facts
- Procedure synonyms: Intracarotid Amytal test
- Procedure definition: Localization of dominant hemisphere for language & memory by injecting sodium amobarbital into the ICA
- Clinical setting triggering procedure: Preoperative workup for temporal lobe epilepsy (TLE)
- Best procedure approach: ICA injection of Amytal on involved side followed by contralateral ICA injection
- Most feared complication: Inadvertent brain stem anesthesia (apnea) due to unrecognized fetal communication of ICA & basilar artery
- Expected outcome: Localization of language & memory predicting possible postoperative deficits

Pre-Procedure
Indications
- Preoperative evaluation in patients with
  - TLE
  - AVM involving eloquent brain
Contraindications
- Fetal communication of ICA & basilar artery
- Uncorrected coagulopathy
Getting Started
- Things to Check
  - Imaging studies & EEG to assess side/location of seizure focus
  - Members of neurology & neuropsychology usually present & perform baseline neurologic exam & EEG
  - BUN, creatinine, PT, PTT, INR
- Equipment List
  - Angiography suite
  - 5 French neuroangiography catheter & 0.035" angled-tip glidewire

Wada Test

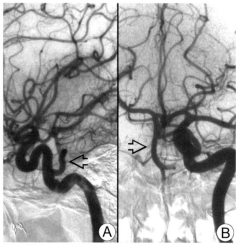

(A) Lateral view of left ICA showing a persistent trigeminal artery (open arrow). (B) AP view, same patient showing marked filling of the basilar artery (open arrow) through this aberrant vessel. A Wada test would require placing a microcatheter in ICA well beyond persistent trigeminal artery (case courtesy Steven Imbesi, MD).

- ▪ Typically young patients & simple hockey-stick catheter will suffice
- o Amobarbital mixed with NS to 10 mg/ml
  - ▪ In consultation with neurology, a predetermined dose (usually 60-90 mg) is drawn through a filter needle into labeled 12 ml syringe

Procedure
<u>Procedure Steps</u>
- Access femoral artery & perform diagnostic angiogram
  - o For TLE the affected side is studied first
  - o Since larger doses (& resultant sedation) are usually needed for testing involved hemisphere with AVM, contralateral side tested first
- Selective catheterization of ICA performed taking care not to cause spasm with wire/catheter
- Exclude fetal communication of ICA & basilar artery
- Assess amount of AComA cross-filling if any
- Patient extends arms & begins counting
- Amytal injected in 1 ml bursts to prevent laminar flow of drug into isolated vascular territory
- Catheter is withdrawn into descending aorta & flushed
- Successful cerebral anesthesia of hemisphere
  - o Contralateral arm weakness
  - o Delta waves noted on EEG
- Speech & memory tested by neurology/neuropsychology
- Wait 30-60 min to allow drug to wear off & repeat procedure for contra-lateral ICA
- Standard post cerebral angiogram orders & patient transferred to recovery

Post-Procedure
Things to Do
- Patients usually observed in PACU 6–8 hrs & discharged if stable & ambulating
- IV normal saline 75–125 cc/hr until patient is taking adequate p.o. fluids

Things to Avoid
- Excessive activity for first 24 hrs
- Lifting > 50 lbs first 48 hrs
- Immersion of puncture site in water x 5 days

Common Problems & Complications
Problems
- Fetal communication of ICA & basilar artery
  o Perform super selective injection with a microcatheter beyond the communication
- PCA also contributes blood supply to hippocampus & is not tested in traditional Wada
- Test is more accurate for language than memory

Complications
- Severe
  o Stroke
  o Brainstem suppression
  o Blindness (use filter needle for Amytal)
- Other complications
  o Carotid dissection/spasm
  o Puncture site complications: Bleeding, dissection, pseudoaneurysm
- Overdose of Amytal (sedation interfering with evaluation)

Selected References
1. Fisher RS et al: Epilepsy for the neuroradiologist. AJNR 18:851-63, 1997
2. Trenerry MR et al: Intracarotid amobarbital procedure. The Wada test. Neuroimaging Clin N Am 5(4):721-8, 1995
3. Wada J: A new method for the determination of the side of cerebral speech dominance: a preliminary report on the intracarotid injection of sodium Amytal in man. Med Biol 14:221-2, 1949

PocketRadiologist™
Interventional
Top 100 Procedures

SPINE & PAIN MANAGEMENT

C1-2 Puncture

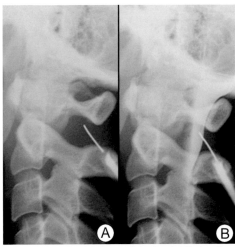

C1-2 puncture for myelography: (A) The needle is placed at the junction of the middle and posterior thirds of the spinal canal. (B) Contrast injection showing the relatively large subarachnoid space (SAS) at C1-2.

Key Facts
- Clinical setting triggering procedure: Myelography above a block or CSF specimen required but LP access difficult or contraindicated
- Best procedure approach: Lateral with patient supine or lateral decubitus
- Most feared complication: Cord/vascular injury

Pre-Procedure
Indications
- LP access for CSF collection difficult or contraindicated
  - o Infection involving lumbar spine/soft tissues
  - o Lumbar epidural hematoma
  - o Lumbar arachnoiditis
  - o Unable to position patient prone or lateral decubitus
- Cervical myelography or myelography above a block

Contraindications
- Absolute
  - o Uncorrected coagulopathy
  - o Obstructive hydrocephalus
- Relative
  - o Congenital craniocervical junction abnormalities such as known Chiari malformation or Klippel-Feil syndrome (review imaging studies)
  - o If myelography is to be performed
    - Severe prior contrast or medication reaction (premedicate)
    - Seizure disorder
    - Seizure threshold lowering drugs: MAO inhibitors, phenothiazines, tricyclics (withhold for 48 hrs prior & 24 hrs following procedure)

Getting Started
- Things to Check
  - o Prior cervical spine imaging studies
  - o CSF volume required to perform requested lab studies

C1-2 Puncture

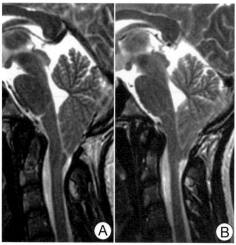

Sagittal T2WIs (A, B) in an asymptomatic patient show findings of classic Chiari I malformation. The SAS at C1-2 is replaced by the low "peg-like" tonsils making C1-2 puncture impossible.

- Equipment List
  - Fluoroscopy with tilt-table or C-arm/angio room
  - Standard myelogram tray
    - 22-gauge 3½ inch spinal needle
  - Nonionic contrast if myelogram is to be performed
    - Iohexol (Omnipaque): 5-10 cc of 180 or 240 mgI/ml
    - Iopamidol (Isovue-M): 5-10 cc of 200 mgI/ml

Procedure
Patient Position/Location
- If performed in fluoro room use a right lateral decubitus position with neutral neck position
  - Place sponge(s) under head so C-spine is perfectly lateral with mandibular rami aligned
- If using C-arm place patient supine (without pillow) or prone and align mandibular rami to assure lateral position
  - Only active neck extension by the patient should be used since cord injury may occur from hyperextension of neck
  - Avoid supine position if contrast is injected (unless head of table can be elevated), otherwise most of contrast will run into head
Procedure Steps
- Localize skin entry site with forceps or metallic marker at junction of middle and posterior thirds of spinal canal
- Betadine & alcohol prep
- Anesthetize skin & subcutaneous tissues with 25-gauge needle & check needle position/trajectory with fluoro
- 25-gauge is exchanged for 22-gauge spinal needle which is advanced with intermittent fluoro toward targeted spot
- SAS 5-6 cm deep to skin in most adults

C1-2 Puncture

- Check frequently for CSF return & rotate needle hub: Dural entry "pop" frequently not detected with C1-2 puncture
- If myelogram is to be performed inject under fluoro to assure subarachnoid needle position

Post-Procedure
Things to Do
- Limit activity for 24 hrs
- Encourage p.o. fluids
- Elevate head 30° for 6 hrs if myelogram performed
- Observe for a minimum of 1 hr prior to discharge
- Patient is given a contact number to call if problems arise

Things to Avoid
- Driving/operating machinery for 24 hrs

Common Problems & Complications
Problems
- If unable to obtain CSF, confirm spine is in complete lateral position & confirm needle is not too posterior
- Dural infolding may occur obstructing CSF flow if neck is extended & therefore a neutral position is preferred
- Epidural venous puncture may occur & usually SAS will be entered upon advancing needle 1-2 mm

Complications
- Severe
  - C1-2 cord injection (closely monitor initial contrast injection)
  - Injury to low-lying vascular structures (PICA)
  - Cord injury from hyperextension of neck (particularly elderly patients), only active neck extension by the patient should be used
  - Seizure (avoid running bolus of contrast into head)
- Other complications
  - Headache much less common in comparison to LP

Selected References
1.   Robertson HJ et al: Cervical myelography: Survey of modes of practice and major complications. Radiology 174(1):79-83, 1990
2.   Burt TB et al: Dural infolding during C1-2 myelography. Radiology 158(2):546-7, 1986
3.   Orrison WW et al: Lateral C1-2 puncture for cervical myelography. Part III: Historical, anatomic, and technical considerations. Radiology 146(2):401-8, 1983

Cervical Discography

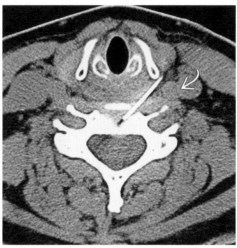

CT guided needle placed into the C4-5 disc. The needle is placed medial to the carotid artery (curved arrow), and lateral to the thyroid lamina.

Key Facts
- Provocative disc injection to evaluate neck and cervical radicular pain
- Performed in the setting of discordant clinical exam and imaging findings
- Anterolateral approach at C3-4 to C6-7 with strict aseptic technique
- Must avoid injury to carotid and vertebral arteries
- Results of procedure helpful in directing medical/surgical therapy

Pre-Procedure
Indications
- Neck and cervical radicular pain with equivocal or conflicting imaging/EMG findings
- Suspected discogenic source of headache (C2-3, C3-4)
- Delineate symptomatic levels prior to cervical fusion
- Continued postoperative radiculopathy (scar vs. disc)
Contraindications
- Uncorrected coagulopathy
- Severe prior contrast or medication reaction (relative-premedicate)
- Local or systemic infection
- Avoid any level with imaging findings of spinal cord compression
Getting Started
- Things to Check
  - Review all pertinent prior imaging studies
  - Review referring physician's history, physical, and clinic notes
  - Perform focused neurological exam
  - Assess patient's baseline pain severity (scale of 0-10) and distribution
- Equipment List
  - C-arm fluoroscopy with filming capability
  - 1% lidocaine
  - 25-gauge spinal needle
  - 3 cc syringes containing nonionic low osmolar contrast (intrathecal safe)

Cervical Discography

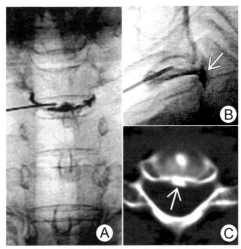

Full thickness annular tear (Grade V): Needle is placed into the disc space via an anterolateral approach (A). Lateral film (B), and CT (C) show contrast (arrows) extending beyond the disc margins (case courtesy Chi-Shing Zee, MD).

- Dilute to 1/3 strength with saline if performing post discography CT
  o Alternatively, may use antibiotic prophylaxis regimen of 1 gram cefazolin in 10 cc sterile saline mixed with 45-50 cc nonionic low osmolar contrast

Procedure
Patient Position/Location
- Supine with neck extended; place roll under shoulders if necessary
- Right anterolateral approach preferred to avoid esophagus (if CT guidance is not used)

Equipment Preparation
- C-arm 30-45 degrees oblique with craniocaudal angulation tangential to disc space being studied

Procedure Steps
- Localize fluoroscopically with skin entry at anterior margin of SCM, and disc entry just medial to uncinate process for levels C3-4 to C6-7
- 25-gauge advanced to disc with right hand while retracting the carotid sheath laterally with left hand
- Check needle position frequently with intermittent AP, oblique and lateral fluoroscopy to avoid vertebral artery and spinal canal
- Gently inject disc until plunger rebounds (usually ≤ 0.5 cc of contrast)
- Document for medical record
  o Injected volume
  o Injection resistance
  o Pain level (0-10)
  o Concordance with usual pain pattern
- Film disc in multiple projections with needle in place
- May obtain limited CT (3 slices parallel to each disc) post procedure

Cervical Discography

Findings & Reporting
- Grading scale for annular tears
  - Grade 0: Normal nuclear anatomy
  - Grade I: Internal fissure involving inner third of annulus
  - Grade II: Involves middle third of annulus
  - Grade III: Involves outer third of annulus = 30° disc circumference
  - Grade IV: Involves outer third of annulus & > 30° disc circumference
  - Grade V: Full-thickness tear with extra-annular leakage

Post-Procedure
Things to Do
- Observe patient for 30 minutes post procedure before discharge
- Ice pack may be applied for 20 minutes to relieve local discomfort
- Patient is given a contact number to call immediately if fever or other systemic signs of infection develop

Common Problems & Complications
Problems
- Cervical disc annular lesions are common on discography and may be coincidental
  - Positive results duplicate usual pain pattern
Complications
- Severe
  - Injury to carotid, vertebral arteries
  - Injury to trachea, esophagus
  - Bacterial or chemical discitis
- Other complications
  - Local pain and odynophagia for 2-3 days

Selected References
1. Siwek SM et al: Discography in clinical practice. In Waldman SD (ed): Interventional pain management 2nd ed. Philadelphia, W.B. Saunders. 135-41, 2001
2. Schellhas KP: Diskography. Neuroimaging Clin 10(3):579-96, 2000
3. Schellhas KP et al: Cervical diskography: Analysis of provoked responses at C2–C3, C3–C4, and C4–C5. AJNR 21: 269-75, 2000

Cervical Facet Injection

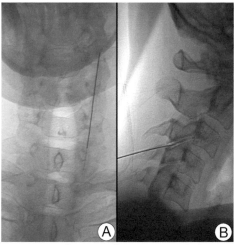

Cervical facet joint injection showing satisfactory intra-articular location of the needle at C 3-4. (A) AP view, and (B) lateral view. The needle was placed from a posterior approach with caudocranial angulation of the needle (case courtesy Chi-Shing Zee, MD).

Key Facts
- Facet blockade accomplished by two techniques
  - Direct intra-articular injection of C3-4 to C7-T1 facets
  - Medial branch block (MBB) of primary posterior ramus of C3 to C7
- Diagnostic &/or therapeutic injection for suspected facet joint syndrome
- Lateral or posterior approach is best for intraarticular injection
  - Lateral best for MBB
- Must avoid injury to vertebral arteries
- May provide long-term pain relief & diagnose source of neck pain

Pre-Procedure
<u>Indications</u>
- Facet joint syndrome
  - Focal paraspinal tenderness worse in the morning
  - Pain upon direct palpation
  - Pain on extension & lateral bending
  - Absence of neurologic deficit
  - May have referred pain to posterior neck & shoulder

<u>Contraindications</u>
- Uncorrected coagulopathy
- Severe prior contrast or medication reaction (relative-premedicate)
- Local or systemic infection
- Avoid glucocorticoids in brittle diabetes, CHF, bleeding gastric ulcers
  - Celestone has least glucocorticoid effect of steroids used

<u>Getting Started</u>
- Things to Check
  - Review all pertinent prior imaging studies
  - Review referring physician's history, physical & clinic notes
  - Perform focused physical exam
  - Assess patient's baseline pain severity (scale of 0-10) & distribution

Cervical Facet Injection

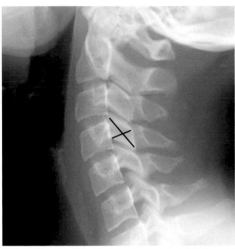

Medial branch block: The midpoint of the lateral mass is targeted via a lateral approach (intersection of lines).

- Equipment List
  - C-arm fluoroscopy with filming capability
  - 1% lidocaine
  - 22 or 25-gauge spinal needle
  - Connecting tubing & 3 cc syringes containing nonionic low osmolar contrast
  - 3 cc syringes with
    - 1:1 mixture of 0.5% Marcaine & steroid (Celestone, Depo-Medrol, or triamcinolone) for therapeutic block
    - 0.5% Marcaine for diagnostic block

Procedure

Patient Position/Location
- Lateral approach: Lateral decubitus position
- Posterior approach: Prone with neck slightly flexed

Equipment Preparation
- C-arm beam parallel to facet joint for lateral approach
- Caudocranial C-arm angulation for posterior approach

Procedure Steps
- Mark skin
  - Lateral approach: Target inferior (posterior) joint capsule
  - Posterior approach: Skin is marked several cm below joint for a "down-the-barrel" needle placement into posterior joint capsule
- After sterile prep & local anesthesia, needle is advanced into joint with intermittent fluoro
  - "Walk" off facet & into joint if bone is contacted with needle
  - Intraarticular location confirmed with 0.25-0.5 cc contrast & then fully aspirated
- 0.5-1.0 cc of Marcaine & steroid injected
  - Avoid administering more than 15 mg Celestone, 100 mg Depo-Medrol, or 80 mg triamcinolone if multiple levels are treated

Cervical Facet Injection

- o Initial course of three monthly injections may be administered & if successful repeated 4-6 times/year
- o Alternatively, if pain responds patient may be eligible for radiofrequency ablation of medial branch nerves
- For MBB central aspect of lateral mass is targeted from lateral approach
  - o Each facet is innervated by medial branch nerves above & below facet requiring 2 MBBs per facet level
  - o Primarily a diagnostic procedure
  - o If pain responds consider radiofrequency ablation of medial branch nerve
- Document for medical record
  - o Pain pattern with initial needle placement & injection
  - o Concordance with usual pain pattern
  - o Pain level (0-10) post injection

Post-Procedure
Things to Do
- Observe patient for 20 minutes post procedure before discharge
- Patient is given a contact number to call immediately if fever or other systemic signs of infection develop

Common Problems & Complications
Problems
- Symptoms often due to multiple factors which may yield conflicting results
- Severely narrowed joints may be difficult to access (perform MBB if unable to enter joint)

Complications
- Severe
  - o Vertebral artery injury
  - o Septic arthritis
  - o Spinal nerve injury
- Other complications
  - o Local pain/numbness at injection site for 24 hrs
  - o Insomnia for 1-2 days secondary to steroids

Selected References
1. Silbergleit R et al: Imaging-guided injection techniques with fluoroscopy and CT for spinal pain management. RadioGraphics 21:927-39, 2001
2. Gray DP et al: Facet block and neurolysis. In Waldman SD (ed): Interventional pain management 2nd ed. Philadelphia, W.B. Saunders. 446-83, 2001
3. Murtagh R: The art and science of nerve root and facet blocks. Neuroimaging Clin N AM 10(3): 465-77, 2000

Cervical Myelogram

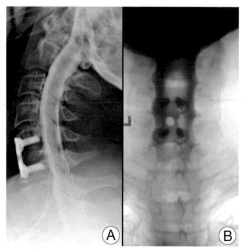

80 year old male with neck pain and bilateral arm radiculopathy. MRI was non-diagnostic due to hardware from a prior discectomy and fusion. Slight posterior indentation of the thecal sac is noted at C4-5, and C6-7 on the lateral view (A). Normal nerve root sleeve filling is seen on the AP view (B).

Key Facts
- Procedure definition: Introduction of myelographic contrast to evaluate cervical cord and nerve roots
- Clinical setting triggering procedure: Neck pain &/or radicular symptoms in patients unable to undergo MRI
- Performed via lumbar or C1-2 approach
- Must avoid nerve/cord injury, injection of material other than intrathecal-safe contrast may result in death
- Remains an important tool for evaluation of cervical disc/foraminal disease & can be performed safely as an outpatient procedure

Pre-Procedure
Indications
- Patient with neck pain &/or radicular symptoms with
  - MRI unsafe implanted devices
    - Pacemakers
    - Cochlear implants
    - Older aneurysm clips
    - Neurostimulators
  - Fixation hardware artifact obscuring area of interest on MR
  - Need for clarification of MRI findings (disc vs. osteophyte)
Contraindications
- Absolute
  - Uncorrected coagulopathy
  - Obstructive hydrocephalus
- Relative
  - Severe prior contrast or medication reaction (premedicate)
  - Seizure disorder
  - Seizure threshold lowering drugs: MAO inhibitors, phenothiazines, tricyclics (withhold for 48 hrs prior & 24 hrs following procedure)

Cervical Myelogram

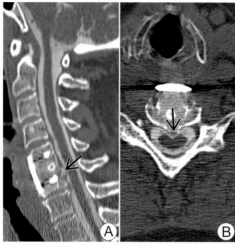

CT myelogram in the same patient. Sagittal reformatted image (A) and axial image (B) show a posterior osteophyte (arrows) and indentation of the cord.

<u>Getting Started</u>
- Things to Check
  - Prior cervical spine imaging studies
  - Lumbar plain films if available & if lumbar approach is to be used
- Equipment List
  - Fluoroscopy room with tilt-table
  - Standard myelogram tray
    - 3½-inch spinal needle: 20 or 22-gauge if CSF is to be collected, otherwise may use 25-gauge (reduces headache risk)
    - 22-gauge preferred for C1-2 puncture
  - Nonionic contrast
    - Iohexol (Omnipaque): 10 cc of 300 mgI/ml for lumbar approach, 5-10 cc of 180 or 240 mgI/ml for C1-2 approach
    - Iopamidol (Isovue-M): 10-15 cc of 300 mgI/ml for lumbar approach, 5-10 cc of 200 mgI/ml for C1-2 approach

Procedure
<u>Patient Position/Location</u>
- Lumbar approach: L2-3 or L3-4 is localized with patient prone
  - Bolster under abdomen widens interspinous space
- C1-2 approach: Right lateral decubitus, target junction of middle and posterior thirds of canal
  - Place sponge(s) under head so C-spine is perfectly lateral
<u>Equipment Preparation</u>
- Low kVp technique
- Shoulder or ankle restraints for support when table is tilted head down
<u>Procedure Steps</u>
- Lumbar approach
  - Prep & drape, removing excess Betadine with rubbing alcohol
  - Anesthetize with 25-gauge needle & reconfirm position with fluoroscopy
  - Interspinous or parasagittal needle placed into thecal sac

Cervical Myelogram

- o Contrast injected over 1-2 min to avoid dilution
- o Needle removed & patient placed in lateral decubitus
- o Tilt table head-down & run contrast into C-spine (side bend neck to keep contrast out of head), then return to prone position
- C1-2 approach
  - o Needle placed into posterior subarachnoid space under fluoroscopy
  - o Contrast & connecting tubing attached
  - o Confirmation of subarachnoid needle position with small amount of contrast injection
  - o 5-10 cc of contrast injected with table in slight reverse Trendelenburg to keep contrast in spine
  - o Remove needle & place patient prone for filming
- Filming: AP, cross-table lateral, and shallow & steep obliques
  - o Swimmer's view for cervicothoracic junction in large patients

Post-Procedure
Things to Do
- CT: Foramen magnum to T2 at 1-2 mm slice collimation & sagittal/coronal reformats (roll patient prior to CT to thoroughly distribute contrast)
- Elevate head 30° for 6 hrs
- Limit activity for 24 hrs
- Encourage p.o. fluids
- Observe for a minimum of 1 hr prior to discharge
- Patient is given a contact number to call if problems arise
Things to Avoid
- Driving/operating machinery for 24 hrs

Common Problems & Complications
Problems
- Lumbar subdural injection avoided by monitoring contrast injection & repositioning needle if free flow of contrast is not obtained
- In patients with advanced lumbar degenerative disease, a parasagittal (interlaminar) approach is preferred
Complications
- Severe
  - o C1-2 cord injection (closely monitor initial contrast injection)
  - o Injury to low-lying vascular structures (PICA)
  - o Cord injury from hyperextension of neck (particularly elderly patients), only active neck extension by the patient should be used
  - o Seizure (avoid running bolus of contrast into head)
- Other complications
  - o Spinal headache seen in up to 20% (limit activity for 24 hrs post myelography & encourage fluids), may require blood patch in persistent headache

Selected References
1. Robertson HJ et al: Cervical myelography: survey of modes of practice and major complications. Radiology 174: 79-83, 1990
2. Shapiro R: Myelography, 4th ed. Year Book Medical Publishers, Inc. 1984
3. Newton TH et al: Modern Neuroradiology, Volume 1. Computed Tomography of the Spine and Spinal Cord. Clavadel Press, 1983

CT Cisternography

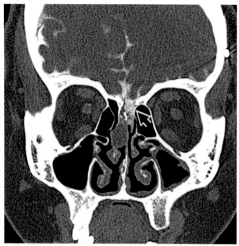

Coronal CT in a trauma patient showing a defect in the cribriform plate, with contrast extending into the left nasal cavity (open arrow).

Key Facts
- Procedure definition: Evaluation of CSF cisterns of brain with intrathecal contrast administration
- Clinical setting triggering procedure: CSF oto- or rhinorrhea
- Contrast administered via a lumbar puncture
- Expected outcome: Demonstration of location of CSF leak for surgical repair

Pre-Procedure
Indications
- Traumatic, spontaneous, or iatrogenic CSF leak in clinical setting of
  - Patients without high-resolution CT demonstrated skull base defects
  - Patients with multiple skull base fractures to direct surgical repair
- Evaluation of cisternal masses
  - In patients unable to undergo MR (i.e. arachnoid cyst vs. epidermoid)
  - To determine if an arachnoid cyst communicates with surrounding CSF
- Search for leaking perineural cyst in spontaneous intracranial hypotension

Contraindications
- Absolute
  - Uncorrected coagulopathy
  - Obstructive hydrocephalus
- Relative
  - Severe prior contrast or medication reaction (premedicate)
  - Seizure disorder
  - Seizure threshold lowering drugs: MAO inhibitors, phenothiazines, tricyclics (withhold for 48 hrs prior & 24 hrs following procedure)

Getting Started
- Things to Check
  - Prior imaging studies
  - Lumbar plain films if available
- Equipment List

CT Cisternography

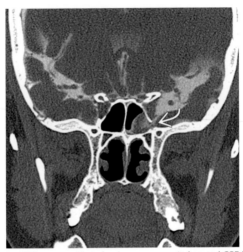

More posterior CT in same patient showing an unexpected second CSF leak arising from the lateral wall of the sphenoid sinus (curved arrow). The demonstration of the additional CSF leak altered the surgical approach.

- o Fluoroscopy room with tilt-table
- o Standard myelogram tray
  - • 3½-inch spinal needle: 20 or 22-gauge if CSF is to be collected, otherwise may use 25-gauge (reduces headache risk)
- o Nonionic contrast
  - • Iohexol (Omnipaque): ~6 cc of 240 mgI/ml
  - • Iopamidol (Isovue-M): ~6 cc of 200 mgI/ml

Procedure
Patient Position/Location
- • L2-3 or L3-4 is localized with patient prone
  - o Bolster under abdomen widens interspinous space
Procedure Steps
- • Prep & drape, removing excess Betadine with rubbing alcohol
- • Anesthetize with 25-gauge needle & reconfirm position with fluoroscopy
- • Interspinous or parasagittal needle placed into thecal sac
- • Needle removed & patient placed in lateral decubitus
- • Tilt table head-down & run contrast cephalad, then return to prone position
- • 30-40° Trendelenburg for 10-20 minutes
- • CT
  - o Rhinorrhea: Coronal & axial 1-2 mm sections through anterior skull base
  - o Otorrhea: Coronal & axial 1-2 mm sections through temporal bones
  - o Soft-tissue and bone algorithm reconstructions
Findings
- • CT demonstrates skull base defect & contrast extending through defect
Alternative Procedures/Therapies
- • Radiologic

CT Cisternography

- o High-resolution CT alone may be sufficient when imaging and clinical findings are concordant
- o MR cisternography (± intrathecal gadolinium) have been described

Post-Procedure
Things to Do
- Elevate head 30° for 6 hrs
- Limit activity for 24 hrs
- Encourage p.o. fluids
- Observe for a minimum of 1 hr prior to discharge
- Patient is given a contact number to call if problems arise

Things to Avoid
- Driving/operating machinery for 24 hrs

Common Problems & Complications
Problems
- Lumbar subdural injection avoided by monitoring contrast injection & repositioning needle if free flow of contrast is not obtained
- In patients with advanced lumbar degenerative disease, a parasagittal (interlaminar) approach is preferred

Complications
- Severe
  - o Seizure
  - o Contrast allergy
- Other complications
  - o Headache
  - o Positional (temporary) increase in CSF leakage

Selected References
1. Jinkins RJ et al: Intrathecal gadolinium-enhanced MR cisternography in the evaluation of clinically suspected cerebrospinal fluid rhinorrhea in humans: Early experience. Radiology 222:555-9, 2002
2. Stone JA et al: Evaluation of CSF leaks: High-resolution CT compared with contrast-enhanced CT and radionuclide cisternography. AJNR 20: 706-12, 1999
3. Drayer BP et al: Cerebrospinal fluid rhinorrhea demonstrated by metrizamide CT cisternography. AJR 129:149-51, 1977

Lumbar Translaminar Steroids

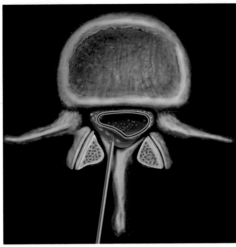

20-guage Tuohy needle is placed with a paramedian, oblique, translaminar approach into the posterior epidural space and steroid is injected.

Key Facts
- Placement of needle thru lamina, into posterior epidural space
- Confirm needle position in epidural space (EDS) by fluoroscopy, contrast injection and loss of resistance
- Localized delivery decreases risk of systemic side effects
- Pain relief, even of short duration may provide significant benefit and facilitate rehabilitation

Pre-Procedure
Indications
- Low back pain especially with lumbar radiculopathy

Contraindications
- Active systemic infection, or infection of skin on lower back
- Cauda equina syndrome
- Severe, poorly-controlled congestive heart failure (CHF)
- Poorly-controlled diabetes mellitus (DM)
- Previous reaction to steroids e.g. psychotic episode
- Uncorrectable bleeding diathesis

Getting Started
- Things to Check
  - Back and leg symptoms
  - CHF, DM, peptic ulcer disease, prior steroid injections, leg edema, previous spine surgery
  - If on heparin or Coumadin
  - INR, PT, platelets, glucose and creatinine
  - Previous MRI and/or CT to help choose target level
- Equipment List
  - 20-gauge Tuohy needle
  - Corticosteroid e.g. triamcinolone or betamethasone
  - Myelogram approved iodinated contrast
  - Preservative free saline and local anesthetic (LA)

Lumbar Translaminar Steroids

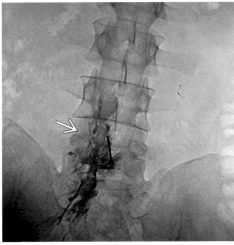

Epidurogram (white arrow) in this patient is predominantly left sided as patient is prone. Contrast injection with fluoroscopy helps show where injectate goes.

Procedure

Patient Position
- Prone

Procedure Steps
- Choose level based on symptoms and MRI findings
  - Look at amount of fat in posterior lumbar epidural space
  - Choose level close to where pain seems to originate and that has a reasonable amount of epidural fat
- Draw up steroid and saline into one syringe
- Typical dosage of triamcinolone is 20-60 mg
- Typical dosage of betamethasone is 6-18 mg
- Add a similar volume of preservative free saline (e.g. 1-3 cc) to syringe and mix with corticosteroid
- LA injection into EDS is optional

Paramedian Oblique Fluoroscopic Approach
- Count lumbar vertebrae
- Choose a level of entry e.g. L4-5 or L5-S1
- Move fluoroscope about 5 to 10 degrees ipsilateral oblique
- Move fluoroscope 5 to 10 degrees caudal
  - Makes needle enter epidural space diagonally
  - Increases relative size of epidural space
  - Because EDS is vertically orientated, and somewhat rectangular
- Position interlaminar space midway between pedicles
- Needle target is posterior midline of interlaminar space
- Put target into center of field of view
  - Helps to minimize parallax
- Magnify target
- Big target easier to hit
- Collimate to about a 5 cm radius around target
- Administer LA subcutaneously
- Superimpose hub of needle over tip

- Advance needle down to ligamentum flava
  - Will have a lot of resistance in ligamentum flava
- Advance very slowly so that entry into EDS is precisely controlled
  - Advancement should be millimeter by millimeter
- Upon passing thru ligamentum flava there is usually an abrupt drop in resistance to needle advancement

Epidurogram
- Confirm needle tip position on lateral and AP view
- Visually confirm that no CSF is flowing out of needle
- Check for loss of resistance by injecting contrast
  - There will be a loss of resistance when EDS is entered
- Check for characteristic epidural distribution of contrast
- Steroid can now be injected into epidural space

Injection Technique
- Inject slowly
  - Can inject thru short length tubing from a myelogram or LP kit
  - Be careful to make sure needle tip is not dislodged
  - Displacement of needle could lead to intrathecal injection
- Periodically watch for washout under fluoro as steroid is injected
  - Washout of previously injected contrast helps confirm still in EDS
- Inquire as to how patient is doing

Post-Procedure
Things to Do
- Monitor blood pressure, pulse and O_2 saturation
- Confirm normal lower extremity strength and movement of feet
- Confirm ambulatory before discharge home in 1 or 2 hours

Common Problems & Complications
- Diabetic patients should be informed blood glucose will be elevated and that medications will need increased dosing
- Steroid "flare" with transient increase in pain
- Epidural hematoma or abscess
- Headache secondary to inadvertent dural puncture
- Complications of steroid such as fluid retention, headache, dysphoric mood, depression, psychotic episode, exacerbation of subclinical infection, hyperglycemia, insomnia and peptic ulcer exacerbation

Selected References
1. Simotas AC et al: Nonoperative treatment for lumbar spinal stenosis clinical and outcome results and a 3-Year survivorship analysis. Spine 25:197, 2000
2. Gundry CR et al: Epidural hematoma of lumbar spine: 18 surgically confirmed cases. Radiology 187:427-31, 1993
3. El-Khoury GY et al: Percutaneous procedures for diagnosis and treatment of lower back pain: diskography, facet-joint injection, and epidural injection. AJR 157:685-91, 1991

Lumbar Discography

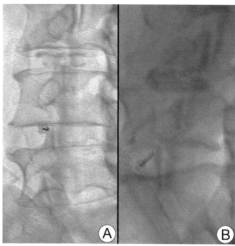

(A) and (B) Posterior lateral approach for lumbar discography with confirmatory AP and lateral views. Oblique view is used to set up approach to disc. Endplates at disc space level are superimposed in straight line. Needle is advanced just anterior to SAP towards nucleus pulposus.

Key Facts
- Procedure definition: Intradiscal injection of iodine contrast to create pressure within disc to try to recreate original pain symptoms
- Clinical setting: Confirmatory test to establish diagnosis of discogenic pain which may be suspected by clinical findings of sitting intolerance, forward flexion intolerance, and possible radiculopathy; imaging may be nonspecific showing more disc abnormalities than clinically relevant
- Best procedure approach
  - Posterolateral - targeting for needle trajectory passing just superior to superior articular process
  - Needle should be placed centrally in the nucleus of the disc as confirmed by AP and lateral fluoroscopic views
  - Alternate approach: Transthecal
- Expected outcome: Diagnosis of discogenic pain

Pre-Procedure
Indications
- Confusing imaging and clinical settings when discogenic pain is suspected
- Pre-surgical fusion
- Post-surgical fusion
- Pre-intradiscal electrothermal therapy or percutaneous disectomy
Contraindications
- Infection
- Uncorrected coagulopathy
- Allergy
Getting Started
- Things to Check
  - Clinical exam: Forward flexion intolerance
  - History

Lumbar Discography

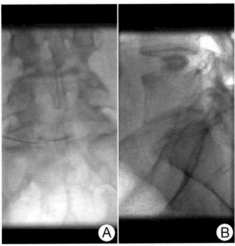

(A) and (B) Demonstrate curved needle trajectory needed for disc entry at L5-S1 where the needle rises over the iliac crest and then inferiorly and medially into the L5-S1 disc.

- Sitting intolerance
- Record original pain pattern (e.g. low back, right buttock, post right thigh, post right calf to right heel)
- Record pain level on a scale of 10
  - MRI or CT: Disc disease
  - Labs: None unless patient coagulopathic or unless infection suspected
  - Consent
- Equipment List
  - C-arm or biplane fluoro
  - 22 or dual needle set up (18-22 gauge)
  - Omnipaque 180
  - Antibiotics (some operators use prophylaxis with 1 gm Ancef IV or equivalent)
  - Sterile pack

Procedure
Patient Position
- Prone
Procedure Steps
- Fluoroscopic targeting
  - Make C arm isocentric (center patient's target in AP plane, then raise or lower patient in lateral plane until target is also centered in lateral plane); this will allow easy rotation around target with target always in center of fluoro image
  - Posterior lateral targeting starting on side opposite clinical symptoms
  - In oblique view, superiorarticular facet (SAP) should bisect disc
  - Local anesthetic
  - Place needle just anterior and superior to SAP in oblique view
  - Advance until tip centered in nucleus (confirm by AP & lateral views)

Lumbar Discography

- If using a coaxial needle system, advance larger needle to edge of disc, then pass smaller diameter needle coaxially into nucleus
- Inject iodine contrast into nucleus, usually about 1 to 2 cc per level (some operators prefer pressure manometer while injecting)
- Record pain responses: Location, distribution, intensity; does the increased pressure aggravate original pain pattern?
- Plan to do at least one normal level for comparison control
- AP and lateral radiographs for documentation
- Remove needle(s); achieve hemostasis, apply Band-Aid
- Post discogram CT scan – 2 or 3 mm cuts angled to each disc space

Alternative Procedures/Therapies
- Radiologic: MRI, CT myelogram

Post-Procedure
Things to Do
- Outpatient recovery 1 hour post discogram and CT scan
- Bed rest 1-3 days at home
- Analgesics

Follow-up
- Phone call 24 hours, 1 week

Things to Avoid
- Heavy lifting
- Excessive bending, sitting, activity, sports for 4-7 days post-procedure

Common Problems & Complications
Problems
- L5-S1 disc: Iliac crest may block direct needle passage
  - Side bend patient & cranial caudal C-arm angulation
  - Curved needle to pass over iliac crest, then down to L5-S1 disc, turning medially into disc
  - Encountering nerve root: Slow down when approaching SAP, be gentle and ready to back off if nerve is contacted with needle tip; instruct patient to say "shock" immediately; apply small amount of local anesthetic and redirect needle tip slightly anterior or posterior: Some operators prefer "docking" needle that has alternate blunt stylet to push nerve out of the way

Complications
- Infection
- Chemical irritation of disc - may produce pain up to 1 week - some operators prefer to dilute Omnipaque 180 to 33% with sterile saline to reduce chance of chemical irritation
- Nerve injury - see above Problems
- Other potential complications
  - Bleeding if patient coagulopathic
  - Allergy
  - Spinal headache - extremely rare with posterior lateral approach

Selected References
1. Guyer RD et al: Contemporary concepts in spine care lumbar discography. Spine 20(18):2048-59, 1995
2. Horton WC et al: Which disc as visualized by magnetic resonance is actually the pain source? Spine 17(65):164-71, 1992
3. Calhoun E et al: Provocation discography as a guide to planning operations on the spine. JBJS 70B:267-71, 1988

Lumbar Facet Joint Injection

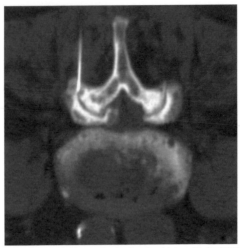

Example of CT guided image for lumbar facet intraarticular injection.

Key Facts
- Procedure definition: Intraarticular injection of anesthetic and/or steroids for pain (usually inflammatory) arising in facet joint
- Clinical setting: Low back pain
  - Often worse in the morning upon awakening
  - Pain typically eases throughout the day
  - Pain worse with hyperextension
  - May be associated with local referred non dermatomal pain
- Best procedure approach
  - Posterior lateral about 10-20°
  - Fluoroscopic or CT guidance
- Most feared complications
  - Very rare
    - Infection
    - Joint capsule injury
- Expected outcome
  - Good short term relief (2 to 3 months)

Pre-Procedure
<u>Indications</u>
- Focal pain arising from facet joint
- Imaging: Degeneration, synovial cyst
<u>Contraindications</u>
- Infection
- Uncorrected coagulopathy
<u>Getting Started</u>
- Things to Check
  - History: Pain worse with prolonged immobilization
  - Physical Exam
    - Focal pain aggravated by direct palpation and correlated with fluoroscopy
    - Worsened pain with hyperextension

Lumbar Facet Joint Injection

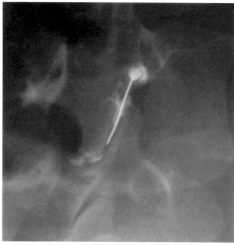

Example of fluoroscopic guided needle entry into the facet joint. Note linear contrast streak within the joint.

- o Imaging: Plain x-rays, CT, MRI
- o Labs: Usually none unless coagulopathy or infection suspected clinically
- o Consent
- Equipment List
  - o Fluoroscope or CT scanner for targeting
  - o 22 or 25-gauge spinal (3-1/2 or longer) needles, 3 cc syringe
  - o Local anesthetic: Lidocaine 1%
  - o Steroid: Depo-Medrol 40 mg
  - o Anesthetic: Marcaine (0.5%)
  - o Non ionic iodine contrast: Omnipaque 180

Procedure
Patient Position
- Prone

Procedure Steps
- Fluoroscopic targeting or CT targeting
  - o 15° to 20° obliquity
- Prep and drape
- Local anesthetic apply to skin and along expected needle course
- 22 or 25-gauge spinal needle directed into joint
- Confirm needle tip position by injecting 0.2 cc iodine contrast (look for linear arthrogram)
- For diagnostic block - inject 0.5 cc Marcaine 0.5%
- For therapeutic block inject (about 0.75 cc) 50/50 mixture of Marcaine 0.5% and Depo-Medrol 40 mg/cc into joint
- Remove needle, apply Band-Aid

Alternative Procedures/Therapies
- Radiologic
  - o Median branch nerve blocks
- Surgical
  - o Facetectomy; fusion

Lumbar Facet Joint Injection

Post-Procedure
<u>Things to Do</u>
- Follow-up 1 week via phone call, then at 4 to 6 weeks depending upon pain level

Common Problems & Complications
<u>Problems</u>
- Hypertrophic spurring - use CT guidance or perform median branch nerve block or try inferior joint entry, bending needle tip may also help
- Synovial cyst - may be drained via sublaminar needle placement using CT guidance

<u>Complications</u>
- Very rare; possible infection, joint capsule injury

Selected References
1. Murtagh FR: Computed tomography and fluoroscopic guided anesthesia and steroid injection in facet syndrome. Spine 13:686-9, 1988
2. Murphy WA: Facet syndrome. Radiology 151:533, 1984
3. Carrera GF: Lumbar facet injection in low back pain and sciatica. Radiology 137:661-4, 1980

Stellate Ganglion Block

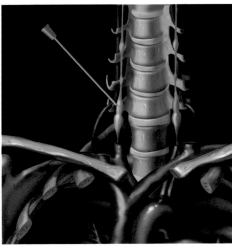

Stellate ganglion is the fusion of the most inferior cervical and most superior thoracic sympathetic ganglia. It is in close proximity to the vertebral artery. The target site is the junction between the transverse process and the lateral body of the C7 vertebra.

Key Facts
- Procedure definition: Image guided needle placement for injection of stellate ganglion with anesthetic or neurolytic
- Clinical setting: Deep somatic pain from upper extremity or head and neck - hyperhidrosis of upper extremity; posttraumatic shock syndrome
- Best procedure approach: Pass needle from anterior to posterior for tip position at junction medial transverse process and lateral aspect of vertebral body (location of superior extent of stellate ganglion)
- Most feared complications
  - Neurologic - stroke
  - Vascular - dissection, vertebral artery bleeding
  - Paralysis of larynx, diaphragm
  - Cardiac - aggravation of CHF
  - Pneumothorax
  - Cardiac or neurotoxicity
- Expected outcome
  - Pain relief
  - Possible Horner's syndrome

Pre-Procedure
Indications
- Pain upper face and neck (e.g. herpes zoster)
- Pain upper extremity (e.g. Raynaud's, chronic arterial emboli, reflex sympathetic dystrophy)
- Post-traumatic shock syndrome
- Hyperhidrosis of upper extremity
Contraindications
- Uncorrected coagulopathy
- Allergy
- Congestive heart failure

Stellate Ganglion Block

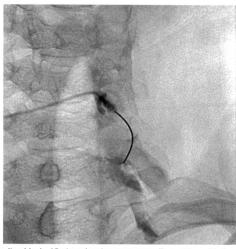

Stellate ganglion block. AP view showing proper needle position with the needle tip at the junction of the transverse process and anterior aspect of the vertebral body. Contrast injection shows no evidence of vascular runoff.

- Contralateral pneumothorax

Getting Started
- Things to Check
  - Pertinent history and physical exam review
  - Labs - none unless patient is coagulopathic
  - Consent
- Equipment List
  - C arm fluoroscope or CT scanner
  - Local anesthetic: 1% lidocaine, 0.25% Marcaine
  - 25-gauge 3-1/2" spinal needle
  - Iodine contrast: Omnipaque 240
  - For neurolysis: Absolute alcohol (arrange general anesthesia)

Procedure

Patient Position
- Prone

Procedure Steps
- Fluoroscope or CT targeting: Junction between anterior lateral aspect C7 vertebral body and proximal ipsilateral transverse process
- Prep and drape
- Local anesthetic (lidocaine 1%) to skin and anticipated needle course
- Direct 25-gauge 3-1/2" spinal needle to above target site, aspirate
- If no blood return, inject 2 cc iodine contrast (Omnipaque 240 or equivalent) under real time fluoro
  - Watch for pooling of contrast locally
  - Watch for any sign of vascular runoff (undesirable)
  - If no vascular contrast runoff
    - Inject long-lasting anesthetic for temporary relief (Marcaine 0.25% 10 cc) slowly; this may need to be repeated on weekly basis for several weeks if reflex sympathetic dystrophy

Stellate Ganglion Block

- Inject absolute alcohol 10 cc slowly for neurolysis (do this with patient under general anesthetic as alcohol is very painful)
- Remove needle, apply direct pressure 5 min; for hemostasis, apply Band-Aid

Alternative Procedures/Therapies
- Surgical
  - Sympathectomy

Post-Procedure
Things to Do
- Monitor patient until stable (usually 30 min) before discharge
- Follow-up
  - 24 hour (by phone)
  - 1 week or as needed in person

Things to Avoid
- Vascular injection

Common Problems & Complications
Problems
- Vascular or subarachnoid communication - watch for these carefully while injecting contrast

Complications
- Intravascular injection: Stroke, neuraxial blocks, cardiac toxicity
- Paralysis of diaphragms and/ or larynx (due to proximity of phrenic nerve and recurrent laryngeal nerve)
- Cardiac block
- Pneumothorax
- Other complications
  - Allergy
  - Bleeding

Selected References
1. Wong W: Management of back pain using imaging guidance. JWI 2(2):88-97, 2000
2. Gangi A et al: Interventional radiologic procedures with CT guidance in cancer pain management. Radiographics 16:1289-304, 1996
3. Erickson SO et al: CT guided injection of the stellate ganglion: Description of technique and efficacy of sympathetic blockade. Radiology 188:707-9, 1993

Celiac Plexus Block

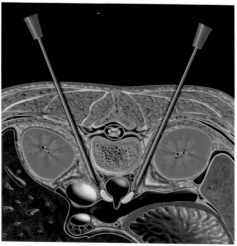

Ganglia are located on either side of the celiac artery just anterior to the aorta and cura of the diaphragms.

Key Facts
- Procedure definition: Injection of anesthetic or neurolytic at celiac sympathetic ganglia located on both sides of celiac artery for control of deep upper abdominal visceral pain
- Clinical setting: Intractable pain from pancreatic cancer, chronic pancreatitis, visceral arterial insufficiency
- Best procedure approach
  - PA: CT guidance - via paraspinous needle trajectory
  - AP: CT or ultrasound-guided needle trajectory via left lobe of liver
- Most feared complications
  - Bleeding
  - Hypotension
  - Pneumothorax
  - Visceral injury
  - Infection
  - Vascular injection
- Expected outcome
  - Pain relief from deep visceral upper abdominal pain

Pre-Procedure
Indications: Intractable Pain from
- Pancreatic cancer
- Chronic pancreatitis
- Visceral arterial insufficiency

Contraindications
- Bowel obstruction
- Uncorrected coagulopathy
- Allergy

Getting Started
- Things to Check
  - Review H & P

Celiac Plexus Block

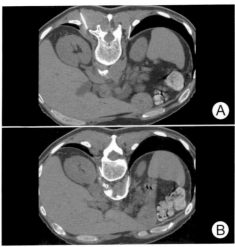

(A) and (B) CT scan demonstrating needle passage very close to the T12 vertebrae such that tips lay anterior to the cura and on either side of the aorta at the level of the celiac artery.

- o Review imaging: CT/MRI, other studies
- o Labs - PT, PTT, INR and platelets
- o Consent
- Equipment List
  - o CT scanner (or ultrasound) for needle guidance
  - o 22-gauge 6 or 8" needles
  - o Iodine contrast (Omnipaque 240)
  - o Local anesthetic: Lidocaine 1% for skin and needle tract; Marcaine 0.25% for temporary ganglion block
  - o Neurolytic: Alcohol (absolute) for more permanent pain relief - (arrange for general anesthetic (GA) if alcohol is used)
  - o Prep kit, drapes
  - o IV set up - have 2 to 3 liters normal saline (ns) available

Procedure
Patient Position
- Prone for posterior to anterior approach (CT guidance)
- Alternative supine for anterior to posterior approach via left lobe liver (CT or ultrasound guidance)

Procedure Steps
- I.V.: NS 100 cc/hr, conscious sedation for temporary block or GA for neurolysis
- Targeting: CT guidance with patient positioned either prone or supine; for prone: Scout view: Start cuts at T12 level - find celiac artery; slight caudal to cranial angulation helps to keep needles out of lungs; US guidance: Target right and left edges of celiac artery
- Local anesthetic to skin and expected needle tract
- For prone patient, direct needles from retro to ante crural position such that tips will lie on both sides of aorta at level of celiac artery

Celiac Plexus Block

- For supine patient - direct needles through left lobe of liver to same location
- Inject 3 to 4 cc iodine contrast - look for local pooling in front of crura of diaphragms adjacent to aorta - (should not be in blood vessel)
- Inject 10 cc Marcaine 0.25% for temporary relief (repeat on weekly basis) or 10 cc absolute alcohol for neurolysis slowly
- Remove needles, apply Band-Aids - watch out for orthostatic hypotension
- Maintain brisk IV fluids for 24 hr.

Alternative Procedures/Therapies
- Narcotics

Post-Procedure
Things to Do
- Admission: Bed rest, IV fluids 24 hrs
- Follow-up: 24 hr - before discharge, 1 week

Things to Avoid
- Celiac block if patient has bowel obstruction
- Bleeding: Use thin 22-gauge or smaller needle, check labs, limit needle passes especially through liver
- Pneumothorax: Use caudal cranial angulation with posterior approach to stay below lungs

Common Problems & Complications
Problems
- Hypotension: Due to blood pooling in visceral vessels; counteract by generous IV fluids and bedrest (24 hr)
- Increased pain if there is bowel obstruction: Due to increased motility of uncontested parasympathetic activity when sympathetics are blocked
- Bleeding: Especially with left lobe of liver
- Pneumothorax

Complications
- Severe
  - Hypotension
  - Bleeding
  - Pneumothorax
- Other complications
  - Bowel perforation
  - Vascular injury
  - Vascular injection

Selected References
1. Waldman SD et al: Interventional pain management. WB Saunders, Philadelphia 360-73, 1996
2. Gimenez A et al: Percutaneous neurolysis of the celiac plexus via anterior approach with Sonographic guidance. AJR 16:1061-3, 1993
3. Matamala AM et al: Percutaneous approach to the celiac plexus using CT guidance. Pain 34:285, 1988

Hypogastric Sympathetic Block

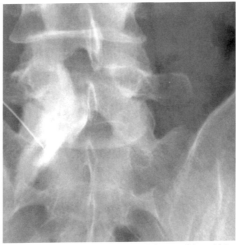

AP view demonstrates posterior to anterior, cranial to caudal, and lateral to medial angulation of the needles which pass over the iliac crest and down into the retroperitoneum just anterior to the L5-S1 disc.

Key Facts
- Procedure definition: Injection of anesthetic or neurolytic at hypogastric sympathetic plexus (located immediately anterior to L5-S1 disc in retroperitoneum for amelioration of deep visceral pain in upper pelvis)
- Clinical setting: Deep visceral pain from
  - Cancer of uterus
  - Cancer of ovaries
  - Prostate cancer
  - Lower bowel cancer
  - Endometriosis
- Most feared complication
  - Intravascular injection: Cardiac/neurotoxicity from Marcaine; vascular injury from alcohol
  - Bleeding
- Expected outcome: Significant pain relief

Pre-Procedure
Indications
- Upper pelvic pain from pelvic malignancy
- Upper pelvic pain from pelvic inflammatory processes e.g., endometriosis
Contraindications
- Uncorrected coagulopathy
- Allergy
Getting Started
- Things to Check
  - Review H&P
  - Labs (Coags if coagulopathy suspected)
  - Consent
- Equipment List
  - C-arm fluoro (or CT scanner)

Hypogastric Sympathetic Block

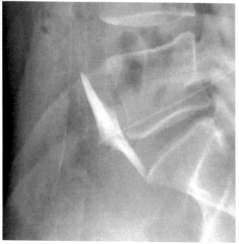

Lateral view showing tip of the needle and normal contrast spread without intravascular communication.

- Local anesthetic (lidocaine 1%, Marcaine 0.25%)
- For neurolysis - absolute alcohol (arrange for general anesthesia)
- Iodine contrast - Omnipaque 240
- Syringes, anesthetic needle, 22-gauge Chiba (6" or 8") needles

Procedure
Patient Position
- Prone

Procedure Steps
- Fluoroscopic targeting - target zone just anterior to L5-S1 disc in retroperitoneum; use slight (15°) obliquity with cranial caudal angulation
- Prep and drape
- Local anesthetic to skin and expected needle tract
- Advance 22-gauge Chiba needle from posterior to anterior over iliac crest from lateral to medial with moderate cranial to caudal angulation so that tip will lay in retroperitoneum anterior to L5-S1 disc
- Aspirate
- Inject (3-4 cc) iodine contrast; check for vascular runoff (undesirable)
- Inject 10 cc 0.25% Marcaine for temporary relief
- Inject 10 cc absolute alcohol for more permanent (requires general anesthesia)
- Remove needles, achieve hemostasis, bandage
- Monitor patient post procedure and discharge when stable (30 min)

Alternative Procedures/Therapies
- Narcotics

Post-Procedure
Things to Do
- Monitor patient (about 30 min) until stable before discharge
- Phone call at 24 hr
- In person at 1 week or as needed

Things to Avoid
• None

Common Problems & Complications
Problems
• Vascular injection
• Iliac crest (Use more cranial caudal angulation)
Complications
• Intravascular injection
• Bleeding
• Visceral perforation

Selected References
1. Waldman SD et al: Interventional pain management. WB Saunders, Philadelphia. 384-91, 1996
2. Pratt RB: Cancer pain. JB Lippincott, Philadelphia. 377-425, 1993
3. Waldman SD et al: Superior hypogastric plexus block using a single needle and computed tomography guidance disruption of a modified technique. Regional Anesthesia 16:286-7, 1991

Impar Ganglion Block

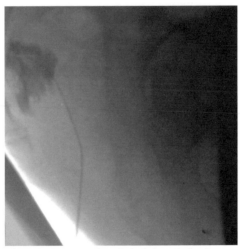

Lateral view demonstrates a curved needle technique starting from a subcoccygeal location to direct the needle posteriorly to the anterior sacral face.

Key Facts
- Procedure definition: Injection of anesthetic or neurolytic at impar ganglion (located in presacral space for control of lower pelvic and perineal pain)
- Clinical setting
  - Pain from lower pelvic/perineal malignancy (e.g., prostate, rectal, uterine cancer)
  - Pain from lower pelvic/perineal inflammatory disease
- Best procedure approach
  - Subcoccygeal
- Most feared complication
  - Infection
  - Bleeding
- Expected outcome
  - Pain relief

Pre-Procedure
Indications
- Lower pelvic perineal pain from malignancy or inflammation
Contraindications
- Uncorrected coagulopathy
- Allergy
Getting Started
- Things to Check
  - Review H&P
  - Labs (coags if coagulopathy suspected)
  - Consent
- Equipment List
  - C-arm fluoroscope
  - Local anesthetic (lidocaine 1%, Marcaine 0.25%)

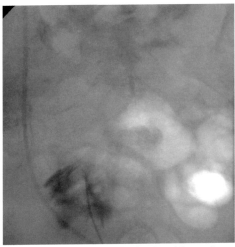

AP view demonstrates midline location of the needle.

- Absolute alcohol for neurolysis - (arrange for general anesthesia)
- Iodine contrast (Omnipaque 240)
- Syringes, anesthetic needles, 22-gauge 3-1/2" spinal needle

Procedure

Patient Position
- Prone

Procedure Steps
- Palpate tip of coccyx
- Bend 22-gauge 3-1/2" needle about 30° in mid section
- Prep and drape
- Local anesthetic to skin site and expected needle tract
- Start 22-gauge just below coccyx immediately direct tip posterior so that it lies in midline just anterior to sacrum
- Inject iodine contrast (2 cc Omnipaque 240) to confirm tip to be in presacral space and not in rectum or in vascular structure
- Slowly inject 10 cc 0.25% Marcaine for temporary relief or 10 cc absolute alcohol for neurolysis
- Remove needle, bandage
- Monitor patient after injection (20 min) to assure stable condition before discharge

Alternative Procedures/Therapies
- Narcotics

Post-Procedure

Things to Do
- Monitor patient (20 min) after procedure or until stable before discharge
- Phone call at 24 hours
- Return visit at 1 week or as needed

Things to Avoid
- None

Impar Ganglion Block

Common Problems & Complications

Problems

- Rectal entry - needle may need to be bent more and driven back posteriorly earlier to reach post rectal (presacral)
- Wandering off midline - check needle position on lateral and AP fluoroscopic views

Complications (Rare)

- Infection
- Bleeding
- Allergy

Selected References

1. Wong W: Management of back pain using imaging guidance. JWI 2(2):88-97, 2000
2. Waldman SD: Interventional pain management. WB Saunders, Philadelphia. 387-90, 1996
3. Karnes LD et al: Effectiveness of an interdisciplinary pain management program for the treatment of chronic pelvic pain. Pain 41:41-6, 1990

Lumbar Median Branch Nerve Block

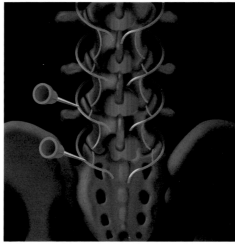

Demonstrates the course of the median branch nerves as they arise from the dorsal nerve roots. Note: That there is dual innervation to each facet joint by median branch nerves arising from above as well as at the level of the joint.

Key Facts
- Procedure definition: Needle placement for blockade of lumbar median branch nerves by anesthetic or percutaneous radiofrequency ablation (PRFA) for pain relief of facet joint pain
- Clinical setting: Refractory pain from facet joints not adequately treated by intraarticular injection
- Best procedure approach
  - Fluoro guided needle placement from posterior to anterior or slight post oblique to anterior direction
- Most feared complications
  - Nerve injury
  - Bleeding
  - Infection
- Expected outcome
  - Months of pain relief

Pre-Procedure
Indications
- Low back pain from facet joint pain
Contraindications
- Allergy
- Uncorrected coagulopathy
- Underlying infection
- Pregnancy
Getting Started
- Things to Check
  - History: Pain worsened with immobility (e.g. upon awakening in the morning), locally referred, not dermatomally radicular
  - Physical exam

Lumbar Median Branch Nerve Block

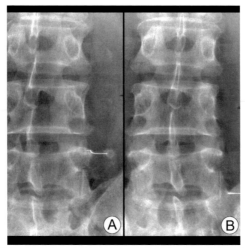

(A) and (B) Demonstrates needle placements for median branch nerve block of the L5-S1 facet.

- Focal tenderness with direct palpation over the facet joint and confirmed by fluoroscopy
- Worsening with hyperextension
- Confirmed by ameliorating pain by anesthetic joint injection
- o MRI or CT
  - Degenerative changes of facet joint
  - Fluid in facet joint
- o Labs
  - Coags if patient on Coumadin or if patient suspected of being coagulopathic
- o Consent
- Equipment List
  - o 22 or 25-gauge spinal needles
  - o C-arm fluoroscope
  - o Local anesthetic: Lidocaine 1% or Marcaine 0.5% (for diagnostic block)
  - o Iodine contrast: Omnipaque 180
  - o PRFA needles, probes PRFA generator (for RF neuroablation)
  - o 3 and 5 cc syringes
  - o Sterile set-up (prep kit, drapes)

Procedure
<u>Patient Position</u>
- Prone
<u>Procedure Steps</u>
- Fluoroscopic targeting
  - o Junction point of medial transverse process and superior articular facet of level at and above the joint involved
  - o Prep and drape
  - o Local anesthetic to skin, sub-cutaneous soft tissues

- o Needle direction: Slight cranial caudal, lateral to medial angulation to target sites
- o For diagnostic block inject 1 cc Marcaine 0.5%
- o For ablation - place PRFA needle tip at target site - confirm proximity to nerve by stimulation test (up to 30 Mz); reposition probe if necessary to ablate: Increase voltage until temperature rises to 43° to 45° c; do 2 cycles of 2 minutes
- o Remove needles
- o Hemostasis, Band-Aids

Alternative Procedures/Therapies
- Radiologic
  - o Facet intraarticular injection
- Surgical
  - o Facetectomy/fusion
- Other
  - o Narcotics, anti-inflammatory medication

Post-Procedure
Things to Do
- Post anesthesia recovery
  - o Observe patient until stable
  - o Analgesics

Follow-up
- 24 hour by phone
- 1 week in person
- 6 month or sooner by phone

Things to Avoid
- None

Common Problems & Complications
Problems
- Not finding nerve during PRFA - (Avoid deep anesthetic)

Complications
- Bleeding
- Allergy
- Infection
- Nerve injury

Selected References
1. Dreyer SJ et al: Low back pain and the zygapophyseal joints. APMR 77:290-9, 1996
2. Bogduck N: Anatomy of so called articular nerves and their relationship to facet denervation in the treatment of low back pain. J Neurosurg 51:172-7, 1979
3. Shealy CN: Percutaneous radiofrequency denervation of the spinal facets. J Neurosurg 43:488-51, 1975

Lumbar Myelogram

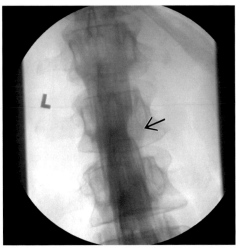

Sequestered disc herniation (arrow) posterior to L2 vertebral body, just above L2-3 disc space. Patient is prone.

Key Facts
- Lumbar myelography involves injection of iodinated contrast into lumbar subarachnoid space (SAS) and obtaining x-rays
  - All myelograms are followed by postmyelogram CT scan
- Most common indication is preoperative evaluation of low back pain in patients unable to undergo MRI or with equivocal MRI
- Most common levels to puncture are L2-3 and L3-4
- Lateral fluoroscopy is helpful to confirm needle is in SAS and not subdural
- Most common complication is spinal headache

Pre-Procedure
Indications
- Low back pain and radiculopathy unable to undergo MRI or equivocal MRI
Contraindications
- Increased intracranial pressure due to mass lesion
- Uncorrectable bleeding diathesis
- Allergic to iodinated contrast and not premedicated with steroids
Getting Started
- Things to Check
  - Bleeding history, platelets, PT, PTT, INR
  - History of previous myelograms or other spinal procedures
  - Previous lumbar spine plain films, CT or MRI if any available
  - History of seizures or medications which may lower seizure threshold
- Equipment List
  - 3½ or 5½ inch (large patients) 22-G spinal needle and myelogram kit

Procedure
Patient's Position
- Prone with head of table elevated about 30 degrees
- Patient should be secured to table with Velcro wrap, arm and foot rests

Lumbar Myelogram

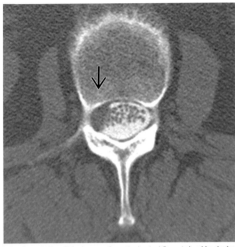

Sequestered disc herniation (black arrow) posterior to L2 vertebral body (same patient).
Note: Mass effect on right side of thecal sac. Patient is supine

- o Instruct patient that head of table will be elevated and lowered

Procedure Steps
- Draw up myelogram approved contrast in 20 cc syringe, connect with long tubing from kit and remove air bubbles
  - o Note number of cc in syringe as will be guide to how much injected
- Count lumbar vertebrae
  - o Usually there are 5 lumbar vertebrae
  - o Counting down from 1st thoracic vertebrae can be helpful
  - o Cephalad angulation of image intensifier (II) helps visualize transitional vertebrae at lumbosacral junction
- Elevate table and move II closer to patient to increase field of view (FOV)
- Obtain AP and lateral scout radiographs of lumbar spine
  - o Include lowermost ribs and upper sacrum on same film
- To obtain "true" AP view, center spinous processes between pedicles
- For "true" lateral view lower lumbar, superimpose bilateral iliac crests
- For "true" lateral of upper lumbar, superimpose bilateral 11th or 12th ribs

Needle Placement
- Blot dry remaining liquid Betadine from patient's back
- Do not want to enter at symptomatic level which is usually L4-5 or L5-S1
  - o Therefore should usually enter at L2-3 or L3-4
  - o Do not enter higher because may hit conus
- Use a paramedian, oblique, translaminar approach
- Move II about 10 degrees caudal and 10 degrees towards you
  - o Put target in center of FOV, magnify and collimate tightly
- Do not touch needle tip with gloves, but if must handle, grasp with gauze
- Superimpose tip and hub and advance towards interlaminar space
- Will encounter increased resistance at ligamentum flavum
  - o Now advance slowly in 2 mm increments
- Make sure hub hatch (and therefore bevel) is turned sideways, i.e. to face right or left as this approach decreases incidence of spinal headache

Lumbar Myelogram

- Will have loss of resistance when enters epidural space and then another loss of resistance when "pops" thru dura to enter SAS

<u>Contrast Injection</u>
- Check for spontaneous return of cerebrospinal fluid (CSF)
- If no flow of CSF, try these options
  - Check AP and lateral fluoro that needle tip in center of spinal canal
  - Further elevate head of table and can rotate needle 90 degrees
- If referral service requested CSF specimen, then collect it now
- Be careful when connect tubing to needle that needle tip not moved
- Typical doses for lumbar myelography in adults are 12 to 14 cc Omnipaque 180
- Contrast injected into SAS should quickly flow downward, away from needle tip, become diluted, and outline cauda equina nerve roots
  - If does not occur, likely are not in the SAS and may be in subdural space (SDS) or epidural space (EDS)
- Injection into EDS is relatively amorphous, and moves slowly
- Injection into SDS tends to collect at tip and nerve roots are not visible
  - Lateral view helpful

<u>Views</u>
- Obtain bilateral oblique, AP and lateral views of the lumbosacral SAS
  - Get magnified, collimated views of lower lumbar levels
- Also obtain AP and lateral views supine and prone of conus region, because lesions here can mimic lesions of lower lumbar levels
  - Contrast will be anterior on prone and posterior on supine views
- Tilting table upright helps fill cul-de-sac and concentrates contrast in lower lumbar SAS
- Standing lateral flexion and extension views can be obtained if table tilts 90 degrees to floor and patient able to cooperate
- These views may be helpful for evaluation of spondylolysis, spondylolisthesis and spinal instability

<u>Post Myelogram CT</u>
- Transport patient to CT scanner with head of bed (HOB) elevated to 45 degrees
- Obtain 2 mm axial sections from mid T12 thru S2 with sagittal and coronal reconstructions

Post-Procedure
<u>Things to Do</u>
- Observe patient 4 hours with HOB elevated at 45-60 degrees
- Encourage hydration and avoid medications which lower seizure threshold

Common Problems & Complications
- Spinal headache-worsens upright and improves recumbent
- Epidural abscess or hematoma
- Nerve root irritation and transient increase in usual pain
- Seizure

Selected References
1. Wildermuth S et al: Lumbar spine: Quantitative and qualitative assessment of positional (upright flexion and extension) MR imaging and myelography. Radiology 207:391-8, 1998
2. Jones SB et al: A transsacral approach through the sacral hiatus for myelography. AJR 169:1179-81,1997
3. Peterman SB: Postmyelography headache: a review. Radiology 200:765-70,1996

Lumbar Puncture (LP)

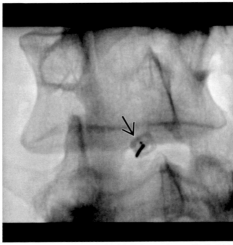

Interlaminar space is placed in center of field of view and magnified. A left paramedian oblique approach is utilized with needle tip superimposed on hub (arrow).

Key Facts
- 22-gauge (G) needle is placed into lumbar subarachnoid space (SAS)
- Main goal is usually to obtain CSF while avoiding traumatic tap
- Most common problems are traumatic tap and spinal headache

Pre-Procedure
<u>Indications</u>
- Meningitis
- Subarachnoid hemorrhage (SAH) with negative CT scan
  - LP is more sensitive that CT for SAH
- Intrathecal chemotherapy
- Pseudotumor cerebri and measurement of opening/closing pressure
- Cytology and flow cytometry in patients at risk for CNS tumor spread

<u>Contraindications</u>
- Increased intracranial pressure due to mass lesion
  - Can check noncontrast head CT in patients at risk
- Platelets less than 50,000 or INR greater than 1.5 (relative CI)
- Infection of skin in planned puncture area
- Critically ill or uncooperative patient may require general anesthesia

<u>Getting Started</u>
- Things to Check
  - Bleeding history, platelets, PT, PTT, INR
  - Any previous LPs or spine surgery such as posterior, lumbar bony fusion
  - Clarify with referral service how much CSF should be obtained and pager number of person from referral service to process specimen
  - Helpful to have an assistant when opening pressure to be obtained
- Equipment List
  - 3½ or 5½ inch (large patients) 22-G spinal needle and LP kit

Lumbar Puncture (LP)

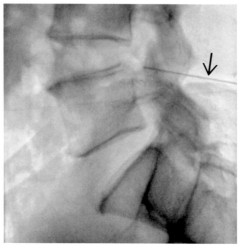

Lateral view of LP with 22-G needle (arrow). To obtain a more accurate lateral view, the iliac crests could be better superimposed. Lateral view helps avoid placing needle too anterior.

Meningitis Precautions
- When patient on meningitis precautions, should be consented on floors or in ER and then sent directly to procedure room

Procedure

Patient Position
- Prone with head of table elevated about 30 degrees

Equipment Preparation
- Connect tubing to side-port of 3-way stopcock
  - Yields faster CSF drainage than connecting tubing directly to needle because apex of tubing loop is lower
- Connect manometer to superior port of 3-way stopcock
- Stand up CSF tubes in numerical order in LP kit

Procedure Steps
- Puncture usually made at L2-3, L3-4 or L4-5
- Blot dry remaining liquid Betadine from patient's back
- Use a paramedian, oblique, translaminar approach
- Target is midpoint of thecal sac
- Move II about 10 degrees caudal and 10 degrees towards you
  - Put target in center of FOV, magnify and collimate tightly
- Do not touch needle tip with gloves, but if must handle, grasp with gauze
- Superimpose tip and hub and advance towards interlaminar space
- Will encounter increased resistance at ligamentum flavum
  - Now advance slowly in 2 mm increments
- Make sure hub hatch (and therefore bevel) is turned sideways, i.e. to face right or left as this approach decreases incidence of spinal headache
  - Places cutting edge of bevel parallel to long axis of dural fibers
- Will have loss of resistance when enters epidural space and then another loss of resistance when "pops" thru dura to enter SAS
- Check for spontaneous return of CSF

Lumbar Puncture (LP)

- If no flow of CSF, try these options
  - Check AP and lateral fluoro that needle tip in center of spinal canal
  - Further elevate head of table and can rotate needle 90 degrees

Opening Pressure
- Table must be flat for measurement of CSF opening pressure
- Opening pressure must be obtained before CSF is collected
- Measure the length of the spinal needle and measure stopcock
  - Need to add this amount to number of cm measured on manometer
- Stopcock should be open only for flow from needle to manometer
- Slight phasicity of the CSF-air interface helps confirm a patent system from thecal sac to manometer
- Now proceed to obtaining CSF
  - Change direction of 3 way stopcock so that CSF in manometer will flow thru side port into collection tube
- In patients with pseudotumor cerebri, check closing pressure after collecting CSF

CSF Collection
- Tipping table further upward can speed CSF flow, but needle may move
- Only put tubing minimal distance into collection tube to facilitate changes
- Position tubing and collection tube so that CSF flows downward steeply
  - A Band-Aid secured to sterile drape can support collection tube
- Put 2 to 4 cc in tube #1 for cell count and chemistry
- Put 4 to 6 cc in tube #2 for microbiology
- Put 8 cc in tube #3 for cytology
- Put 2 to 8 cc in tube #4 for cell count and other tests

Intrathecal Chemotherapy
- Use AP and lateral fluoro to confirm needle in center of thecal sac
  - This is safest site for injection of intrathecal chemotherapy
- Check again for spontaneous return of CSF before injecting chemotherapy

Post-Procedure
- Encourage hydration and supine positioning for 1 to 4 hours

Common Problems & Complications
- Delay processing of CSF causes cell lysis and possible inaccurate cytology
- Traumatic tap can be significant problem as may lead to false positive diagnosis of SAH and may make CSF cell count and protein unreliable
  - Main thing to avoid is anterior epidural venous plexus
  - Lateral fluoroscopy can be helpful to avoid anterior spinal canal
  - Consider repuncture at a higher lumbar level
  - Can occur with good technique as intrathecal vein is variably present
  - Blood may clear between tubes #1 and #4
- Epidural abscess or hematoma
- Nerve root irritation and transient increase in usual pain
- Spinal headache-worsens upright and improves recumbent
  - Usually resolves spontaneously with supine positioning
  - May require epidural blood patch
- Tonsillar herniation and death

Selected References
1. Yousry I et al: Cervical MR Imaging in Postural Headache: MR Signs and Pathophysiological Implications AJNR 22:1239-50, 2001
2. Peterman SB: Postmyelography headache: a review. Radiology 200:765-70, 1996

Lumbosacral Selective Nerve Block

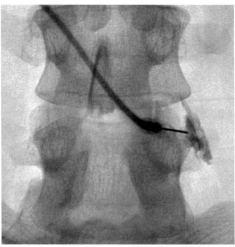

The exiting nerve root passes out of neural foramen to cross anterior to the mid section of the next lowest transverse process. Contrast outlining the nerve root as the needle had been placed just along the superior margin of the next lower transverse process to encounter the nerve root.

Key Facts
- Procedure definition: Image-guided needle placement for application of anesthetic to nerve or for ablation of nerve by neurolytic agent or pulsed radiofrequency
- Clinical setting
  - Uniradicular pain
  - For diagnosis of pain origin
  - For therapy of radiculopathy
- Best procedure approach
  - Post ganglionic approach for diagnostic block
  - Periganglionic (transforaminal) for therapeutic block
- Most feared complications
  - Nerve injury
  - Anesthetic communication with subarachnoid space
- Expected outcome is pain relief

Pre-Procedure
Indications
- Uniradicular pain
- Painful neuroma
- Alternative application of steroids to epidural space foramina (e.g. due to post-surgical scarring)

Contraindications
- Uncorrected coagulopathy
- Contralateral pneumothorax (with high lumbar nerve block)
- Allergy
- Superficial infection along path of needle
- Pregnancy

Getting Started
- Things to Check

Lumbosacral Selective Nerve Block

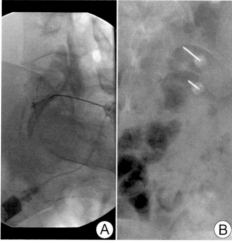

(A) Needle position is at the 6:00 position of the rostal pedicle for transforaminal epidural steroid injection (AKA periganglionic nerve block). (B) Demonstrates sacral posterior foramina where needles would be targeted for sacral nerve blocks.

- History and physical exam: Determine distribution of pain e.g. which dermatome
  - Imaging - MRI and/or CT - check for a stenotic lesion such as osteophyte or disc
  - Labs - usually none unless coagulopathy suspected
  - Consent
- Equipment List
  - Imaging system: C-arm fluoroscopy unit or CT scan
  - Local anesthetic: Lidocaine 1%, Marcaine 0.5%
  - 22 or 25-gauge spinal needles (3-1/2" inch)
  - Iodine contrast: Omnipaque 180 or 240
  - Steroid: Celestone 6 mg/cc or Depo-Medrol 40 mg/cc
  - Sterile pack - prep and drapes

Procedure
<u>Patient Position</u>
- Prone
<u>Procedure Steps</u>
- Image targeting
  - Postganglionic lumbar diagnostic nerve block PA view - target mid section superior margin inferior transverse process
  - Periganglionic - slight 10°-15° obl; PA approach - target 6:00 position of pedicle (superior margin of neural foramen) for periganglionic (aka. transforaminal epidural steroid injection)
  - Sacral nerve block - target posterior sacral neural foramina
- Prep and drape
- Local anesthetic to skin and along expected needle path
- Under image guidance direct needle to target - warn patient of possible paresthesia - be ready to back off needle 2 mm at that moment

Lumbosacral Selective Nerve Block

- Inject 2 cc iodine contrast to outline nerve sheath and look for epidural spread (with periganglionic or sacral nerve block - change needle position slightly if vascular communication is seen
- For diagnosis - inject 2 cc of 1% lidocaine
- For therapy inject 1 cc Celestone (6 mg/cc) – or 1cc Depo-Medrol (40mg/cc) with 1 cc Marcaine 0.25%
- Remove needle
- Hemostasis, apply Band-Aid

Alternative Procedures/Therapies
- Radiologic
  o Epidural steroid injection
- Surgical
  o Foraminotomy
- Other: Pulsed radiofrequency ablation

Post-Procedure

Things to Do
- Patient may leave when stable
- Follow-up in 1 week

Things to Avoid
- Should not drive if there is transient motor or sensory deficit
- For transforaminal (periganglionic) injection - needle tip should not go more medial than medial border of pedicle

Common Problems & Complications

Problems
- Vascular communication and/or subarachnoid space entry - avoid by visualizing with real time fluoroscopy while injecting contrast
- Unable to reach foramen - try bend at tip of needle to rotate or skin into neuroforamen

Complications
- Severe
  o Nerve injury - avoid by being gentle when approaching expected position of nerve - be ready to back off - don't inject contrast into nerve; inject around it
  o Bleeding
  o Vascular filling - toxic systemic
  o Subarachnoid space effect filling
  o Paralysis
- Other complications
  o Allergy

Selected References
1. Zennar OH et al: Periganglionic foraminal steroid injections performed under CT control. AJNR 19:349-52, 1998
2. Weiner BK et al: Foraminal injection for lateral lumbar disc herniation. JBJS 79:804-7, 1997
3. Waldman S: Atlas of interventional pain management. WB Saunders, Philadelphia. 297-9, 1988

Lumbosacral Caudal Steroids

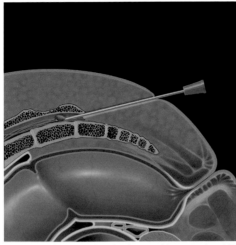

20-gauge needle is placed into sacral epidural space with a posterior midline approach. Contrast is injected to confirm needle location in lateral and AP planes and then steroid is injected.

Key Facts
- Typically provides good bilateral injectate distribution
- This is an alternative to S1 approach
- Advantages of caudal approach
  - Landmarks remain intact after spine surgery
  - Increased distance of needle from thecal sac
  - Steroid can be delivered close to S1 nerves
- Disadvantages of caudal approach
  - Difficult to reach higher lumbar levels with injectate

Pre-Procedure

Indications
- Low back pain especially with lumbar radiculopathy
- Previous lumbar spine surgery e.g. with posterior bony fusion

Contraindications
- Active systemic infection or infection of skin on lower back
- Poorly controlled CHF or DM

Getting Started
- Things to Check
  - Obtain relevant history and physical examination
  - Back and leg symptoms
  - CHF, DM, peptic ulcer disease, prior steroid injections, leg edema, previous spine surgery
  - INR, PTT, platelets, glucose and creatinine
  - Previous MRI and/or CT and check sacrum for Tarlov cysts
- Equipment List
  - Corticosteroid e.g. triamcinolone or betamethasone
  - Myelogram approved iodinated contrast e.g. 3 to 5 cc
  - Preservative free saline (PFS) and local anesthetic (LA)
  - 20-gauge Touhy needle is usually used

Lumbosacral Caudal Steroids

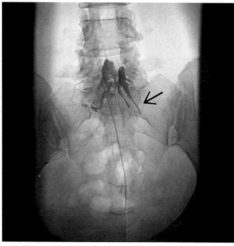

Caudal approach for injection of epidural steroid. Note: Epidurogram shows contrast extending out thru right S1 sacral foramina (arrow).

o Can use 18-gauge Tuohy to speed up procedure when necessary

Procedure

Patient Position/Location

- Prone
- Several pieces of 4 x 4 gauze should be placed into upper gluteal fold to minimize spillage of Betadine down onto perineum

Procedure Steps

- Choose level based on symptoms and MRI findings
- Draw up corticosteroid, PFS and local anesthetic
  - o Place them in color coded or different size syringes
  - o Typical dosage of triamcinolone is 20-60 mg
  - o Typical dosage of betamethasone is 6-18 mg
  - o Add similar volume of PFS (e.g. 1-3 cc) and mix with steroid
- Increased injectate volume helps increase distance of distribution
- LA injection into EDS is optional

Needle Placement

- Fluoroscopy unit is placed in lateral view with visualization of skin and sacral canal on same view to facilitate placement of needle
- Palpate sacral cornu and define midline
- Place hemostat on skin in midline below S5 level and check position for skin entry relative to sacral canal
- Magnify target and collimate
- LA is administered subcutaneously and along planned tract
- Needle is advanced in midline, cephalad and anterior at a 30 to 45 degree angle, into sacral canal at S5 level
- If patient complains of shooting pain in leg, withdraw needle a few mm and adjust course slightly
- Once near sacrococcygeal ligament, advance needle in small, controlled increments of about 2 mm at a time
- Usually needle will meet with resistance and then "pop" into sacral canal

- o "Pop" felt as passes thru sacrococcygeal ligament
- Hub may need to be retracted downward to align needle better with long axis of sacral spinal canal
- Needle should be advanced to upper S4 level
- While needle often contacts anterior wall of sacral spinal canal, this is not essential and can be painful
- Check for a lack of CSF or blood return
- Maintaining needle below lower margin of S3 vertebra helps prevent puncture of thecal sac
- Inject contrast to confirm tip is within epidural space
  - o Should be confirmed in lateral and AP plane
- Observe spread of contrast to determine if moves adequately cephalad to target level of likely pain generator

Injection Technique
- A total volume of 10 to 15 cc is recommended to help injectate reach desired level such as L4-5 or L5-S1
- An epidural catheter can be advanced within sacral canal to reach more cephalad EDS
- Patient may have discomfort in buttock and leg during injection which quickly fades when injection is halted

Post-Procedure
Things to Do
- Monitor blood pressure, pulse and O2 saturation
- Confirm normal lower extremity strength and movement of feet
- Confirm ambulatory before discharge home

Common Problems & Complications
- Diabetic patients should be informed blood glucose will be elevated and that medications will need increased dosing
- Increased pain of intermediate duration
- Epidural abscess or hematoma
- Spinal headache secondary to inadvertent dural puncture
- Complications of steroid such as fluid retention, dysphoric mood, depression, psychotic episode, exacerbation of subclinical infection, hyperglycemia, insomnia and peptic ulcer exacerbation, headache
- Suboptimal distribution of injectate
- Small hematoma of periosteum can cause pain
- Urinary retention in elderly male with baseline obstructive condition, due to local anesthetic

Selected References
1. Simotas AC et al: Nonoperative treatment for lumbar spinal stenosis clinical and outcome results and a 3-Year survivorship analysis. Spine 25:197, 2000
2. Gundry CR et al: Epidural hematoma of lumbar spine: 18 surgically confirmed cases. Radiology 187:427-31, 1993
3. El-Khoury GY et al: Percutaneous procedures for the diagnosis and treatment of lower back pain: diskography, facet-joint injection, and epidural injection. AJR 157:685-91, 1991

Needle Control

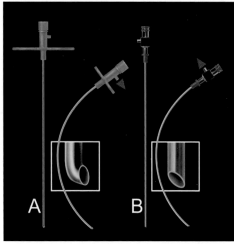

Tuohy needle (A) moves in same direction as bevel and hub ridge. Therefore, bevel is placed on concave side of curve with bowed needle technique. Spinal needle (B) moves in direction opposite of bevel and bevel is put on convex side of curve.

Key Facts
- Needle control refers to techniques for steering needles during fluoroscopic procedures
- These techniques are most important for spinal injection procedures such as epidural steroid injection and discography
  - These techniques are also useful for other procedures such as percutaneous nephrostomy
- Spinal needles move in direction opposite of their bevel
- Tuohy needles move towards their bevel
- For virtually all spinal injection procedures it is important to clearly define needle target, magnify it and to place it in center of field of view (FOV)

Pre-Procedure
Indications
- Spinal injection procedures
- Percutaneous nephrostomy
- Other procedures that require steering a needle with fluoroscopic guidance towards a well defined target

Contraindications
- Depends on specific procedure

Getting Started
- Things to Check
  - Bleeding history, platelets, PT, PTT, INR
  - History of symptoms and if any previous surgery in region of planned procedure
  - Check previous imaging studies
- Equipment List
  - Spinal needles are used for majority of spinal injection procedures
  - Tuohy needles are used for translaminar lumbar epidural steroid injection

Needle Control

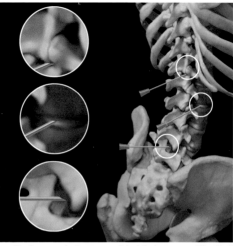

Uppermost needle shows posterior approach to inferior recess of facet. Middle needle shows oblique lateral approach for discography. Lowest needle shows translaminar approach for epidural steroid injection.

Procedure

Patient Position

- Prone positioning is utilized for most spinal injection procedures
- Slight elevation of one side towards a decubitus position can facilitate obtaining a lateral view for some procedures such as discography

Procedure Steps

- Target for needle placement is chosen e.g. nucleus pulposus for lumbar discography
- Line up fluoroscope with planned path of needle
  - o Allows needle hub and tip to be superimposed and advanced in a straight line to a large extent
- Put target in center of FOV
  - o Helps to minimize parallax
- Magnify as much as possible
  - o Bigger targets are easier to hit
- Collimate
  - o Minimizes radiation exposure

Bevel Control Technique

- Line up needle with fluoroscopic beam
- Superimpose hub over tip as this helps for guiding needle in a straight line
- Spinal needles will move in direction opposite of their bevel
- The bevel is on same side as "ridge" or "rectangular bump" or "hub hatch" that is seen on plastic hub of needle stylet
- Therefore spinal needles will move opposite ridge on stylet
  - o Thus by using ridge as a guide, needle can be steered
- This allows needle to be steered as advanced without withdrawing it from skin
- It is helpful to advance needle in small increments, so if goes off course, will be easier to redirect

Bowed Needle Shaft Techniques
- This technique is more powerful than bevel control
- Enables epidural steroid injections, discograms and lumbar punctures in large patients to be performed quickly
- Midshaft of spinal needle is bowed with convexity on side of hub ridge
- This accentuates needle movement in direction opposite bevel and hub ridge
- For right-handed physicians, the hub is held with right hand and left hand holds needle just distal to apex of needle curve
  - Right hand on hub steers tip to optimal alignment
  - Left hand then advances needle in small increments

Bent Needle Technique
- Distal 2 cm of spinal needle can be bent about 10-20 degrees away/opposite from hub ridge
- Use a piece of sterile gauze to bend needle tip
  - Do not touch needle with gloves as powder from gloves may get on needle
- Needle will move away from hub ridge
- Needle advancement is same as with bevel control concept
- The difference is that needle tip of spinal needle now moves further in direction opposite hub ridge

Post-Procedure
Things to Do
- Routine post-procedure management

Common Problems & Complications
- Pain
- Bleeding
- Inability to advance needle to desired location
- Inadvertent puncture of subarachnoid space

Selected References
1. Johnson BA et al: Epidurography and therapeutic epidural injections: Technical considerations and experience with 5334 cases. AJNR 20:697-705, 1999
2. Dreyfuss P: The power of bevel control. International Spinal Injection Society (ISIS) newsletter 3:16, 1998

Sacroiliac Joint Injections

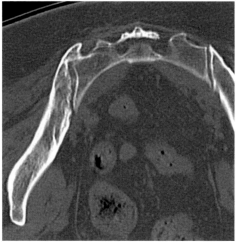

CT showing fusion of the left SI joint posteriorly. The right SI joint is well seen, and a medial to lateral needle trajectory would facilitate joint entry.

Key Facts
- Procedure definition: Placement of pain-relieving medications (anesthetic and steroids) by injection into the SI joint
- Clinical setting
  - Focal pain at SI joint
  - Stiffness in the morning upon awakening or after prolonged sitting
  - Local referred nondermatomal pain common
  - Positive Patrick's, Gaenslens tests
- Best procedure approach: CT or fluoro-guided needle placement posterior to anterior, slight medial to lateral needle angulation to inferior most aspect of joint
- Most feared complication (rare): Infection, allergic reaction
  - Expected outcome: Positive pain relief

Pre-Procedure
<u>Indications</u>
- Painful sacroiliac joint usually due to degenerative or posttraumatic etiology

<u>Contraindications</u>
- Underlying infection
- Uncorrected coagulopathy

<u>Getting Started</u>
- Things to Check
  - Medications that might cause patient to be coagulopathic
  - Underlying infection
- Equipment List
  - Fluoroscopy (or CT)
  - Iodine contrast (Omnipaque)
  - Steroids (Depo-Medrol)
  - Anesthetic: Lidocaine (1%) for skin and soft tissues, Marcaine (0.5%) for joint

Sacroiliac Joint Injections

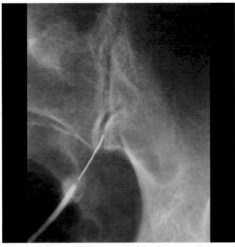

Proper needle position in the inferior aspect of the SI joint. Note: Medial to lateral and inferior to superior needle trajectory.

o 22 or 25-gauge 3-1/2" needle

Procedure
Patient Position
- Patient Position
  o Prone

Procedure Steps
- Fluoroscopic or CT targeting of inferior joint margin
- Prep and drape
- Local anesthetic - lidocaine 1%
- Needle trajectory typically posterior to anterior, slight medial to lateral
- Inject 1cc iodine contrast to confirm that needle is intraarticular (linear contrast streak)
- Inject 40 mg Depo-Medrol (or equivalent) and 2 cc 0.5% Marcaine

Alternative Procedures/Therapies
- Radiologic
  o Pulsed radiofrequency L5 median branch nerve, S1-S2 dorsal nerves
- Surgical
  o Fusion
- Other
  o Oral pain medicine

Post-Procedure
Things to Do
- Follow-up
  o 1 week by phone
  o 4 to 8 weeks by return visit depending upon pain

Sacroiliac Joint Injections

Common Problems & Complications
<u>Problems</u>
- Iliac bone overlapping SI joint may hinder easy access when using fluoroscopy
  - Try slight bend at tip of needle
  - Try rotating fluoroscope a few degrees back and forth to superimpose anterior and posterior joint openings
  - Target most inferior aspect of joint
  - Or use CT for guidance

<u>Complications</u>
- Very rare - possible infection

Selected References
1. Wong W: Management of back pain using imaging guidance. JWI 2:88-97, 2000
2. Dreyfus P et al: Sacroiliac joint injection techniques in physical medicine and rehabilitation. Clinics of North America 6:4, 1995
3. Laslett M et al: The reliability of selected pain provocation tests for sacroiliac joint pathology. Spine 19:124-9, 1994

Lumbar Spine Biopsy

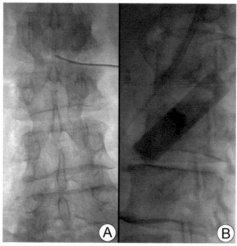

Postero-lateral approach for disc (A) and transpedicular bone (B) biopsies.

Key Facts
- Procedure definition: Obtaining samples of abnormal tissues of the spine, discs, paraspinous soft tissues by needle placement under imaging guidance
- Clinical setting: Suspicion of infection or neoplasm, indeterminate by imaging
- Best procedure approach
  - Transpedicular for bone
  - Costovertebral (parapedicular for bone)
  - Posterolateral for disc or soft tissues
- Most feared complications
  - Bleeding
  - Nerve damage
  - Infection
- Expected outcome
  - Sampling of diagnostic quality

Pre-Procedure
Indications
- Indeterminate vertebral, disc, paravertebral abnormality discovered on imaging
- Differentiate benign from malignant vertebral compression fracture
- Isolate organism for culture and sensitivity in case of treated but persistent osteomyelitis
- Marrow collection for assessment of progression of leukemia during therapy

Contraindications
- Uncorrected coagulopathy
- Uncooperative patient

Getting Started
- Things to Check
  - Physical exam and history

Lumbar Spine Biopsy

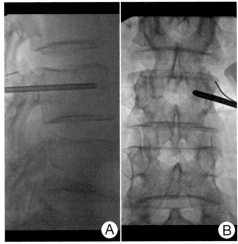

(A) and (B) Demonstrate trajectory and course for transpedicular bone biopsy similar to vertebroplasty.

- o Imaging: Plain film, CT, MRI, bone scan, other studies
- o Labs – PT, PTT, INR, platelets
- o Consent
- Equipment List
  - o Local anesthetic, lidocaine 1%, anesthetic needle (1-1/2 to 3-1/2" 25 gauge)
  - o Bone core biopsy needles - 11 to 17-gauge for bone samples
  - o 22 or 20-gauge Chiba or Crown needles for disc, paraspinous soft-tissue biopsies
  - o Cope trocar catheter drainage systems for abscess pockets
  - o C-arm fluoroscopy or CT scanner for bone or disc biopsies; CT scanner for paraspinous soft-tissue biopsies or for difficult anatomy
  - o Scalpel
  - o Mallet
  - o Sterile pack, drapes

Procedure
Patient Position
- Prone

Procedure Steps
- CT or fluoro targeting based upon suspicious target area on prior imaging
- For disc biopsy, use posterolateral approach similar to discogram to enter slightly lateral to superior articular facet
- For vertebral body biopsy, use transpedicular or parapedicular (costovertebral) approach
- Prep and drape
- Local anesthetic skin to target
- Conscious sedation
- Obtain biopsy samples
- Have pathology preview for adequacy
- Remove needles

Lumbar Spine Biopsy

- Pressure at site for hemostasis
- Steri-strip, bandage

Alternative Procedures/Therapies
- Surgical
  - Surgical excision

Post-Procedure
Things to Do
- Postanesthesia recovery
  - Bed rest, observation 2 to 3 hours
  - Analgesics
  - Discharge when clearly stable

Follow Up
- 24 hour phone call
- 1 week as needed

Things to Avoid
- Keep biopsy entry sites dry 3 days

Common Problems & Complications
Problems
- Patients already on antibiotics may have delayed or no growth of their biopsy specimens, so best to biopsy lesions before patient is placed on antibiotics or wait 1 week after stopping antibiotics
- Biopsy of vascular metastasis (melanoma, renal, thyroid)
  - May need either transarterial embolization prior to biopsy or intraosseus Gelfoam or alcohol embolization through needle at end of biopsy

Complications
- Severe
  - Nerve injury
  - Bleeding
  - Infection
  - Death
- Other complications
  - Allergy

Selected References
1. Wong W: Common spine interventions: Percutaneous biopsies. ASNR Proc 36:107-9, 1998
2. Parker SH et al: Needle biopsy techniques. Radiol Clin North Am 33:1171, 1995
3. Babu NV et al: Computed tomographically guided biopsy of the spine. Spine 19:2436-42, 1994

Lumbar Sympathetic Block

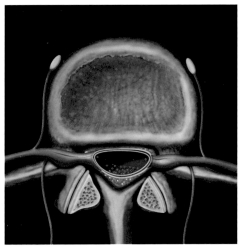

The lumbar sympathetic chain runs from L5 to L2 along the anterior lateral aspect of the lumbar vertebrae.

Key Facts
- Procedure definition: Injection of anesthetic or neurolytic at cranial extent of lumbar sympathetic chain (L2 level) for deep somatic pain arising from lower extremity
- Lumbar sympathetic chain runs from L5 to L2 along the anterolateral aspects of the adjacent vertebrae
- Clinical setting
  - Pain for arterial insufficiency (e.g., Raynaud's, chronic arterial emboli)
  - Pain from reflex sympathetic dystrophy (RSD)
  - Phantom limb pain
  - Hyperhidrosis
  - Posttraumatic syndromes
- Best procedure approach
  - Posterior to anterior with lateral to medial needle angulation
- Most feared complications
  - Intravascular injection
  - Vascular injury
  - Bleeding
  - Ureteral injury
- Expected outcome: Pain relief; breaking cycle of RSD

Pre-Procedure
<u>Indications</u>
- Lower extremity pain from RSD, chronic arterial emboli, arterial insufficiency
- Phantom limb pain
- Pain from lower extremity frostbite, gangrene
- Hyperhidrosis
<u>Contraindications</u>
- Uncorrected coagulopathy

Lumbar Sympathetic Block

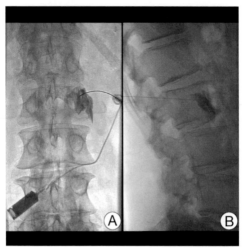

(A) and (B) Demonstrate correct needle placement for lumbar sympathetic blockade (contrast distribution in the retroperitoneum, with no contrast filling of vascular structures).

- Allergy

Getting Started
- Things to Check
  - o Review H&P
  - o Labs (coags if patient suspected of coagulopathy)
  - o Consent
- Equipment List
  - o C-arm fluoro (or CT scanner)
  - o Local anesthetic: Lidocaine 1%, Marcaine 0.25%
  - o For neurolysis - absolute alcohol (arrange for general anesthesia)
  - o Iodine contrast: Omnipaque 240
  - o Syringes, anesthetic needles, 22-gauge (Chiba) needles (6 or 8")

Procedure
Patient Position
- Prone

Procedure Steps
- Fluoroscopic targeting: Anterolateral aspect L2 vertebra
- Prep and drape
- Local anesthetic to skin and along expected needle tract
- Advance 22-gauge needle from patient's back (starting about 3" lateral to midline) to anterior lateral aspect of L2 vertebra
- Aspirate
- Inject iodine contrast (3-4 cc) under real time fluoro - (look carefully for vascular communication)
  - o Iodine contrast should pool in retroperitoneum
- Inject 10 cc Marcaine 0.25% for temporary relief
- Inject 10 cc absolute alcohol for more permanent relief (requires general anesthetic)
- Remove needles, achieve hemostasis - apply bandage

Lumbar Sympathetic Block

- Monitor patient post procedure - discharge when stable (usually 30 min)

Post-Procedure
Things to Do
- Monitor patient (about 30 minutes) after procedure until stable before discharge
- Phone call at 24 hours
- In person at 1 week - Note: For RSD repeat lumbar sympathetic blocks should be done on a weekly basis with Marcaine for usually several weeks

Things to Avoid
- Vascular injection
- For RSD, patient should not remain sedentary but should undergo physical therapy (weight bearing) to break RSD cycle

Common Problems & Complications
Problems
- Vascular injection - avoid by injecting a bolus of 3-4 cc iodine contrast rapidly while fluoroscope is turned on to see if there is vascular communication (brief angiogram)
- Nerve root encounter - avoid by starting slightly cephalad to advance needle superior to transverse process staying cephalad to neuroforamen

Complications
- Intravascular injection
- Bleeding
- Ureteral injury
- Visceral perforation

Selected References
1. Wong W: Management of back pain using imaging guidance. JWI (2):88-97, 2000.
2. Walman SD: Interventional pain management. WB Saunders, Philadelphia. 353-9, 1996
3. Cousins MJ et al: Neurolytic lumbar sympathetic blockade: Duration of denervation and relief of rest pain. Anesth Intensive Care 7(2):121, 1979

Thoracic Myelography

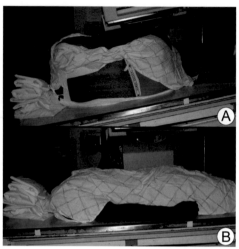

(A) Lateral decubitus position to allow contrast to flow from lumbar to thoracic (but not cervical) region. Lateral view of thoracic spine taken as contrast column is balanced out. (B) AP view obtained by turning patient supine, keeping contrast out of neck and head by balancing patient's position and tucking the head anteriorly.

Key Facts
- Procedure definition: Intrathecal placement of iodine contrast for diagnosis of diseases affecting the thecal sac
- Clinical setting: Diagnosis of pathology either internally within the thecal sac or externally affecting the thecal sac may be used when the patient cannot be evaluated by MRI (e.g. spinal instrumentation, pacemaker, neurostimulator) or in conjunction with MRI for added information often about the adjacent bone or spinal instrumentation which may not be as well imaged on MRI
- Best procedure approach
  - Midline interspinous process - below L2-3
  - Translaminar below L2-3
  - Contrast must be positioned in thoracic region by gravity flow
- Most feared complication
  - Spinal headache
  - Infection
  - Nerve damage
  - Seizure
- Expected outcome = Diagnostic evaluation of thoracic thecal sac

Pre-Procedure
Indications
- Patients with back pain, radiculopathy or other suspected pathology involving or affecting the thecal sac and who cannot be evaluated by MRI
- Above patients with have undergone MRI but require further evaluation
- Evaluation of subarachnoid catheter if morphine induced granuloma is suspected
- Workup for vascular malformation

Thoracic Myelography

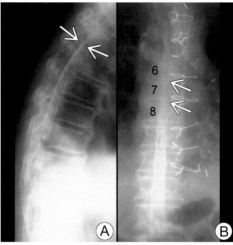

(A) and (B) Demonstrate thoracic myelogram where there is a mid-thoracic extradural block (arrows) from metastatic disease.

Contraindications
- Allergy
- Uncorrected coagulopathy

Getting Started
- Things to Check
  - History, focused physical
  - Labs none unless coagulopathy suspected
  - Review available imaging
  - Informed consent
- Equipment List
  - Fluoroscopy - tilt table
  - Local anesthetic: Lidocaine 1%
  - Spinal needle (20-25 gauge)
  - Intrathecally approved iodine contrast (e.g. Omnipaque 240)

Procedure

Patient Position
- Prone

Procedure Steps
- Fluoroscopic targeting for lumbar puncture
- Prep and drape
- Local anesthetic
- Lumbar puncture: Midline, paramedian translaminar below L2-3 level
- Inject iodine contrast 12-14 cc Omnipaque 240 - pool contrast in lumbar area by positioning patient semi upright
- Roll patient onto lateral decubitus - tip head of table downwards while head is side bent upwards opposite decubitus side
- Allow contrast to flow from lumbar into thoracic area & level out table before contrast reaches cervical subarachnoid space
- Obtain lateral fluoroscopic or overhead radiographs while patient is in lateral decubitus position

Thoracic Myelography

- Turn patient to supine position with head flexed & raise or lower head of table to position contrast in selected portions of thoracic subarachnoid space
- Obtain AP views with overhead tube
- Alternate to lateral decubitus positioning to mobilize contrast is to keep patient prone - Tip head downwards steeply - Raise 1 hip to accentuate flow of contrast into thoracic area - Keep head hyperextended - To keep contrast out of head

Alternative Procedures/Therapies
- Radiologic
  - o MRI if not contraindicated

Post-Procedure
Things to Do
- Post myelographic CT scan
- 5 mm thick by 5 mm interval or thinner from mid C7 to L1
- Post procedure
  - o Bed rest with head elevated 30° x 24 hours
  - o Force p.o. fluids
  - o Avoid phenothiazines
  - o Follow-up
    - ▪ Phone call 24 hours

Things to Avoid
- Ionic and other non-intrathecally approved iodine contrast agents should never be placed in the thecal sac
- Also be careful to control contrast when positioning contrast column from lumbar to thoracic subarachnoid space

Common Problems & Complications
Problems
- Injection in epidural or subdural space (contrast may not flow freely and appear as linear irregular streak when needle is not subarachnoid)

Complications
- Headache (spinal leak)
- Seizures
- Allergy

Selected References
1.   Grossman R et al: Neuroradiology The Requisites. Mosby, St. Louis. 17-9, 1994
2.   Shapiro RL: Yearbook Med Pub, Chicago, 1975
3.   Peterson HO et al: Introduction to Neuroradiology, Harper and Row, Hagerstown. 198-239, 1972

Vertebroplasty

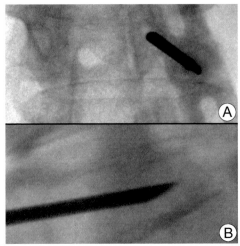

AP (A) and lateral (B) views showing proper transpedicular needle position in a mid-thoracic compression fracture. The needle is advanced to the anterior ¼ of the vertebral body (B).

Key Facts
- Procedure definition: Internal injection of polymethylmethacrylate (bone cement) by injection into painful vertebral compression fracture (VCF)
- Clinical setting: Pain due to VCF that occurs with minimal trauma or spontaneously due to underlying osteoporosis or osteolytic metastasis
- Best procedure approach
  - Transpedicular
  - Parapedicular for small pedicles in upper thoracic
- Most feared complications
  - Neurologic
    - Paralysis
  - Radiculopathy
  - Pulmonary embolus
- Expected outcome
  - Significant reduction in pain often within hours

Pre-Procedure
Indications
- Painful VCF
- Painful osteolytic metastasis
- Painful hemangioma
- Kummels disease
Contraindications
- Absolute
  - Underlying infection
  - Uncorrected coagulopathy
  - Non painful VCF
- Relative
  - Retropulsion (Neurological compromise)
  - Allergy

Vertebroplasty

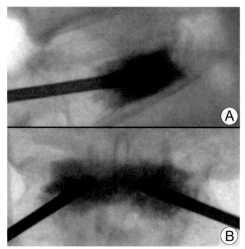

Lateral (A) and AP (B) views showing bipedicular application of cement in this lumbar compression fracture. The cement is confined to the anterior 2/3 of the vertebral body.

- o Severe vertebra plana
- o Fracture posterior vertebral body
- o Acute trauma (possibly associated posterior element fractures)

Getting Started
- Things to check
  - o Physical exam and history
  - o MRI
  - o Check for edema, retropulsion
  - o Labs: Coags
  - o Consent signed by patient
- Equipment List
  - o C-Arm Fluoro
  - o Local anesthetic
  - o 11-gauge or 13-gauge needles
  - o 40 cc PMMA (bone cement), mixing bowl, 1cc moromer
  - o Opacifier: Sterile barium 6 gm
  - o Injection device
    - 1 cc luerlock syringes
    - Injection devices: Various vendors (Parallax, Cook, Stryker, Spinal Specialties)
  - o Mallet
  - o Sterile pack
  - o Antibiotics: Ancef 1 gm IV given 30 min prior to procedure; alternative: Tobramycin 1.2 gm added to cement

Procedure
Patient Position
- Prone
- Hyperextended: Arms folded around head and taped

Vertebroplasty

Procedure Steps
- IV antibiotics IV: 1 gm Ancef 30 min prior to procedure
- Fluoroscopic targeting of pedicles
- Prep and drape
- Local anesthetic, conscious sedation
- Needle placement
  - o Upper outer aspect of pedicle: Oblique enface view
  - o Next lateral view to seat needle with tip at anterior 1/4 of vertebral body
- Mix bone cement, add opacifier (30% by weight - sterile barium)
- Slowly inject cement under real time fluoroscopy filling from anterior to posterior to fill to posterior 1/3 of vertebral body
- Remove needles
- Achieve hemostasis by direct pressure
- Steri-strip and bandage entry sites
- Move patient off of table when ex vivo cement sample hardens

Post-Procedure
Things to Do
- Post anesthesia recovery
  - o Bed rest 3 to 4 hours
Follow-up
- 24 hrs
- 1 week or as needed
- Osteoporosis care (referral to internist)
Things to Avoid
- Avoid getting entry site wet for 4 days post procedure
- Avoid heavy lifting for 6 weeks

Common Problems & Complications
Problems
- Avoid breaching medial or inferior endplates
Complications
- Severe
  - o Paralysis
  - o Nerve injury
  - o Pulmonary embolus
  - o Infection
  - o Death
- Other complications
  - o Allergic reaction
  - o Rib fracture

Selected References
1. Wong W et al: Is intraosseous venography a significant safety measure in performance of vertebroplasty? JVIR 13(2):137-8, 2002
2. Mathis JM et al: Percutaneous vertebroplasty: A developing standard of care for vertebral compression fractures. AJNR 22:373-81, 2001
3. Jensen ME et al: Percutaneous polymethylmethacrylate vertebroplasty in the treatment of osteoporotic vertebral body compression fractures. AJNR 18:1897-904, 1997

PocketRadiologist™
Interventional
Top 100 Procedures

GENITOURINARY

Kidney Biopsy

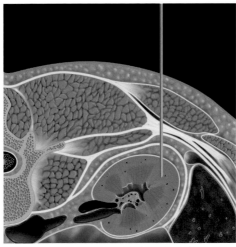

18-guage biopsy needle is placed into renal cortex to obtain core specimen.

Key Facts
- Goal is to obtain core specimen with glomeruli from renal cortex

Pre-Procedure
Indications
- Diffuse disease and abnormal function in native kidney (K)
- Diffuse disease and abnormal function in transplant kidney
- Some renal masses
- Most large renal carcinomas have a characteristic appearance on CT and are surgically removed

Contraindications
- Uncooperative patient (consider general anesthesia)
- Uncorrectable bleeding diathesis
- Severe hypertension is a relative contraindication

Getting Started
- Things to Check
  - Bleeding history, INR, PT, PTT, CBC, BUN, creatinine
  - Obtain type and screen for blood
  - Do not start procedure until have confirmed good IV access e.g. 18 gauge
  - Check if previous CT of abdomen available
  - Check which kidney appears larger and more superficial
  - Check if there is a retrorenal spleen or colon
  - Call pathology to help process and evaluate specimens
    - Increases yield
- Equipment List
  - Use best ultrasound machine available
  - 2-3.5 megahertz ultrasound probe
  - Ultrasound transducer needle guide
  - 18-gauge biopsy gun

Kidney Biopsy

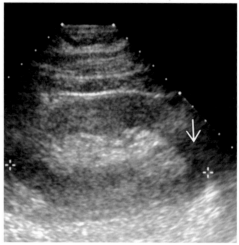

Typical path of biopsy needle into lower pole of kidney (white arrow), the goal is to obtain core specimen with glomeruli from renal cortex.

Procedure
Patient Position
- Prone for biopsy of native kidney
- Supine for biopsy of transplant kidney
- 2 L O2 nasal cannula is commonly given
- Monitor blood pressure, oxygen saturation and pulse

Imaging Guidance
- Ultrasound is most common modality used
- Needle guides that attach to transducer are very helpful
- On rare occasion that indication is mass lesion, CT scan is preferred for imaging guidance
- Downside of CT is that core biopsy guns are bulky and often do not fit into bore of CT scanners

Target with Native Kidneys
- Lower pole of kidney
- Goal is to obtain core specimen with glomeruli from renal cortex

Target with Renal Mass Lesions
- Goal is to place needle into mass lesion
- 22-gauge needle may be adequate
  - o Less risk of bleeding

Technique with Native Kidneys
- Area over kidney is prepped and draped
- Lower pole of kidney is visualized with ultrasound
- Transducer needle guide is lined up with lower pole cortex
- Be generous with local anesthetic at skin and along tract
  - o IV sedation with fentanyl and midazolam is often necessary
- 18-gauge biopsy needle is threaded thru needle guide
- Patient asked to hold breath and needle advanced into lower pole
  - o When needle is in kidney, will move with respirations
- Position of needle tip prior to firing is chosen based on throw length of needle

Kidney Biopsy

- o Goal is to obtain tissue from renal cortex
- o Slotted part of needle should be in renal cortex when needle gun is fired
- Specimen is teased off biopsy needle and given to pathology
- Usually 3 or 4 specimens are obtained
- Ultrasound is then used to check for any evidence of bleeding

Technique with Transplant Kidneys
- Upper pole of kidney is target and patient is supine

Post-Procedure
Things to Do
- Apply firm pressure over biopsy site for 10 minutes
- Observe patient for a minimum of 6 hours
- Some nephrologists routinely admit patient for 23 hours observation and obtain serial hemoglobin levels
- Check blood pressure, pulse, urine output and inquire regarding back pain q 15 min x 2, q 30 min x 2, q 1 hour x 4
- Notify MD if any changes

Common Problems and Complications
- Hematuria is usually not significant and clears within 48 hours
- Blood is like food coloring in that a few drops can redden a large amount of urine
- If blood is forming clots and seems profuse, monitor patient extra carefully and check serial hemoglobins
- If patient develops increasing pain or a change in vital signs, repeat complete blood count should be drawn and period of observation extended
- Consider obtaining a CT scan to check for bleeding
- Incidence of bleeding complications has decreased with trend towards 18 gauge needles instead of 14-gauge
- If bleeding rapidly, platelet transfusion, or transcatheter embolization may be necessary
- Vasovagal reaction
- Subcapsular hematoma and perirenal hematoma
- Retroperitoneal hematoma
- Renal artery pseudoaneurysm and arteriovenous fistula
- Hydronephrosis due to ureteral obstruction by blood clot
- Worsening renal function secondary to obstructive hydronephrosis, or compressive subcapsular hematoma
- Injury to nontarget organs such as liver, spleen and lung
- Pneumothorax

Selected References
1. Cluzel P et al: Transjugular versus percutaneous renal biopsy for the diagnosis of parenchymal disease: Comparison of sampling effectiveness and complications. Radiology 215:689-93, 2000
2. Lechevallier E et al: Fine-needle biopsy of renal masses with CT guidance. Radiology 216:506-10, 2000
3. Pokieser PR et al: Renal biopsy: In vitro and in vivo comparison of a new automatic biopsy device and conventional biopsy systems. Radiology 186:573-6, 1993

Percutaneous Nephrostomy

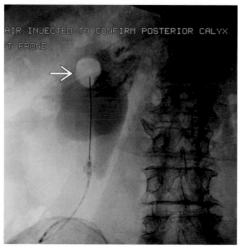

Several cc of air (white arrow) injected into renal collecting system to confirm within a posterior, nondependent calyx. It is important to confirm that needle not in blood vessel prior to injection of air.

Key Facts
- Placement of drainage tube into renal collecting system
- Posterior and lateral calyces are needle target

Pre-Procedure
<u>Indications</u>
- Obstructive hydronephrosis
- Access for antegrade ureteral stent
- Access for percutaneous nephrolithotomy
- Diversion of ureteral fistulae

<u>Contraindications</u>
- Platelets less than 75,000
- Uncooperative patient (consider general anesthesia)

<u>Getting Started</u>
- Things to Check
  - Bleeding history, INR, PT, PTT, CBC, BUN, creatinine
  - Order prophylactic antibiotics
  - Study pre-procedure ultrasound and or CT scan carefully
  - Choose target calyx for entry
  - If for stone removal, choose an approach that will facilitate percutaneous lithotripsy which requires direct contact with stone
    - Usually a middle pole, posterior or lateral calyx is best target for routine nephrostomy and for renal pelvis stones
    - If stone extends into a posterior or lateral infundibulum, then try to go into associated calyx
  - Do not start procedure until have confirmed good IV access
    - Patient can quickly become septic and require IV
- Equipment List
  - Nephrostomy kits contain 21 G entry needle, 0.018" wire, coaxial dilator, 0.035" wire, and metal stiffener in some

Percutaneous Nephrostomy

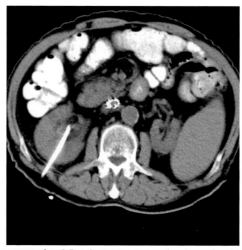

Typical appearance of an 8 French percutaneous nephrostomy placed into the right kidney. Note: If the same approach were used on the left kidney, the spleen could be lacerated.

- o Coaxial dilator with inner part for 0.018" wire and outer part for 0.035" wire
- o 65 cm long, 5 French, hockey stick type tip catheter e.g. Berenstein
- o 0.035" angled tip glidewire and 75 cm long, Amplatz, extra stiff guidewire
- o 8 French nephrostomy with locking loop

Procedure
Patient Position/Location
- Prone
Procedure Steps
- Obtain scout radiographs of kidney and bladder
  - o Be generous with local anesthetic
  - o IV sedation with fentanyl and or midazolam usually necessary
- Use ultrasound or radiopaque anatomical landmarks such as stones seen on a previous CT scan or IVP to plan approach
- Try to initially enter collecting system with a 21 G needle
  - o If proves difficult, switch to an 18 G needle, because easier to steer
- Upon entering system, inject contrast to opacify and evaluate entry site
- Contrast goes preferentially into anterior calyces
- If completely in the collecting system and not at all intravascular, can inject 5 cc of air to increase visualization of posterior nondependent calyces
  - o If entry site acceptable, thread in guidewire
- If decide to enter different site, keep initial needle in place for repeat contrast injections
- Place coaxial dilator over 0.018" wire and then exchange for 0.035" wire
- Manipulate 0.035" guidewire until goes into pelvis and then ureter
  - o If trouble steering, place hockey tip catheter over wire
  - o May also need 0.035 angle tip glidewire to steer into renal pelvis

Percutaneous Nephrostomy

- Place hockey tip catheter over wire and into ureter
- Exchange for Amplatz, extra stiff 0.035" wire to provide support
  - Dilate tract to desired size
- Prepare nephrostomy by flushing all components
- Metal stiffener increases pushability of nephrostomy tube
- Advance nephrostomy over Amplatz wire
- Advance metal stiffener up to parenchyma-calyceal margin, but no further
- Metal stiffener will experience loss of resistance when passes from parenchyma into calyx
- Fix stiffener, and advance nephrostomy into renal pelvis
- Check that distal loop in renal pelvis and not ureter
- Twirl nephrostomy catheter about 90 degrees clockwise or counterclockwise
  - This often helps to form distal loop of catheter
- Activate string lock mechanism of distal loop
- Inject contrast to confirm in location and obtain radiograph
  - Limit contrast if urine purulent or patient septic
- Distal loop should usually be placed in renal pelvis
- With severe hydronephrosis, may pull into a dilated calyx
- Suture catheter to skin with 3-0 monofilament nylon suture

Post-Procedure
Things to Do
- Observe patient at least 6 hours
  - Because if bleeding or urosepsis occur, will usually be evident in this time frame
- Check blood pressure, pulse, urine output and inquire regarding back pain q 15 min x 2, q 30 min x 2, q 1 hour x 4
- Notify MD if any changes
- Then record urine output q shift
- Nephrostomy to gravity drainage
- Flush nephrostomy with 10 cc sterile saline q 2 hours x 2, q 4 hours x 1 and then q 8 hours until urine becomes clear

Common Problems & Complications
- Leakage of urine around tube or from catheter connectors
- Catheter dislodgement and occlusion
- Hematuria usually not significant and will clear in 48 hours
- Blood is like food coloring in that a few drops can redden a large amount of urine
- If blood is forming clots and seems profuse, monitor extra carefully and check serial hemoglobins
- If bleeding rapidly, an arteriogram might be necessary for transcatheter embolization
- Renal subcapsular hematoma can be evaluated with a CT scan

Selected References
1. Millward SF: Percutaneous nephrostomy: A practical approach. JVIR 11:955-64, 2000
2. Gray RR et al: Outpatient percutaneous nephrostomy. RJ 1998:85-8,1998
3. Barbaric ZL et al: Percutaneous nephrostomy: Placement under CT and fluoroscopy guidance. AJR 169:151-5, 1997

Ureteral Stent

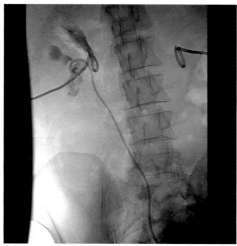

Right percutaneous nephrostomy and antegrade ureteral stent as well as left nephrostomy placed to treat bilateral distal ureter obstruction due to malignancy. Left obstruction not traversable and therefore ureteral stent not placed.

Key Facts
- In general, "ureteral stent" refers to an antegrade internal stent
  - It is a plastic tube, usually 6-10 French
  - Connects renal pelvis to urinary bladder
  - Has sideholes and an endhole at both ends
- Ureteral obstruction is most common indication

Pre-Procedure
<u>Indications</u>
- To bypass a ureteral obstruction due to tumor or stone
- To facilitate ESWL and maintain ureteral patency
- Treatment of ureteral stricture or ligation
- Unsuccessful attempted retrograde ureteral stent

<u>Contraindications</u>
- Frank urosepsis due to ureter obstruction
  - In this situation it is best to establish initial drainage by nephrostomy

<u>Getting Started</u>
- Things to Check
  - If patient has a nephrostomy
  - Coagulation labs
  - Previous abdominal CT if any
    - Look for stone or tumor
- Equipment List
  - 8 French ureteral stent
    - 22 cm long for average height patients
    - 24 cm long for tall patients
  - 9 French peel away sheath
  - 0.035", angled tip, 150 cm long glidewire
  - 0.035", Amplatz, extra stiff 145 cm guidewire
  - 65 cm long, 5 French, hockey-tip catheter

Ureteral Stent

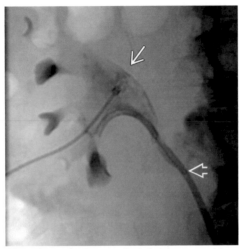

The "pusher" (arrow) is used to keep proximal stent (open arrow) in renal pelvis as string is removed.

Procedure
Patient Position
- Prone

Equipment Preparation
- Flush all components with saline
- Insert pusher into stent

Procedure Steps
- Obtain scout films of kidney and bladder
- Do nephrostogram through indwelling nephrostomy
- Use catheter and glidewire to steer past obstruction
- Place catheter into bladder and inject contrast to confirm in bladder
- Exchange for Amplatz extra stiff wire and place into bladder
- Flush ureteral stent again
  - If not flushed, pusher has a tendency to stick
  - Can cause major delay
- Place ureteral stent over Amplatz wire into bladder
  - Place far into bladder
  - Can always pull it back later
  - Whereas can be difficult to advance later

Positioning the Proximal End
- Make sure inner plastic stiffener is kept within renal pelvis so that it will prevent stent from being pulled out when cut and remove string
- Withdraw proximal end of stent until in renal pelvis
- Keep guidewire thru pusher and proximal stent
- Cut the string which is attached to renal end of stent
- While maintaining guidewire thru stent and forward pressure on proximal stent with pusher, withdraw string
- Must use pusher to keep inward pressure on stent, or stent will be pulled out of kidney
- Can be difficult to withdraw string
  - Vibrating motion of hand pulling on string can be helpful

- o Do not leave string in collecting system as can be nidus for stone formation
- Once string removed, guidewire can be pulled out of ureteral stent, and withdrawn into pusher which is still in renal pelvis

Replacing the Nephrostomy
- Now readvance guidewire further into renal pelvis, so that a nephrostomy can be placed over this wire
- A percutaneous nephrostomy is then placed into renal pelvis
- Obtain spot film to document location of nephrostomy and stent

Alternative Procedures and Therapies
- Radiologic
  - o Nephroureteral stent is a single device which combines the function of a nephrostomy and an antegrade ureteral stent
- Surgical
  - o Retrograde ureteral stents are usually placed by urologists thru a cystoscope

Post-Procedure
Things to Do
- Typically, patient is brought back to interventional radiology suite within 1 to 3 days
- Nephrostogram is obtained by injection of contrast thru nephrostomy
- Purpose of nephrostogram is to check that ureteral stent is patent
- If ureteral stent is patent, then nephrostomy is usually removed
- Stents should be replaced every 4 to 6 months

Complications
- Stent obstruction
- Stent calcification and stone formation
- Stent infection and urosepsis
- Ureter perforation
- Injury to kidney
- Minor or massive bleeding
  - o May require transcatheter embolization
- Bladder irritation and pain
  - o Although usually mild and often temporary, may require removal of stent

Selected References
1. Cockburn JF et al: Radiologic insertion of subcutaneous nephrovesical stent for inoperable ureteral obstruction. AJR 169:1588-90, 1997
2. Yeung EY et al: Percutaneous fluoroscopically guided removal of dysfunctioning ureteral stents. Radiology 190:145-8, 1994
3. Baere TD et al: Ureteral Stents: exchange under fluoroscopic control as an effective alternative to cystoscopy. Radiology 190:887-9, 1994

PocketRadiologist™
Interventional
Top 100 Procedures

CHEST

Lung Biopsy CT Guided

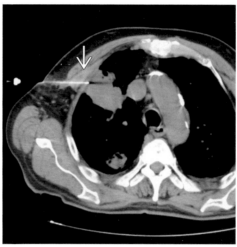

Fine needle (white arrow) biopsy of right lung mass. Note: Needle enters pleural-based component of mass so that risk of pneumothorax is diminished.

Key Facts
- Evaluate previous CT scan to determine best approach
- Consent for both lung biopsy and chest tube
- Adjust needle in soft tissues outside chest until course is correct
  - Then advance into lung mass
- Pathology service should be present

Pre-Procedure
Indications
- Lung mass

Contraindications
- No safe approach
- Uncooperative patient

Getting Started
- Things to Check
  - Prior CT scan of chest
  - Determine if should be supine, prone or decubitus for biopsy
  - Someone in vicinity able to place chest tube
  - Reserve time in CT scanner
- Equipment List
  - 22-gauge, 9 cm long Franseen biopsy needle, works well
  - Other types of needles can be used
  - If 22-gauge unsuccessful, can try 20-gauge
  - Have chest tube available

Consent
- Consent for biopsy and possible chest tube

Procedure
Choice of Imaging Modality
- Large masses can often be biopsied with fluoroscopy, which is fastest method

Lung Biopsy CT Guided

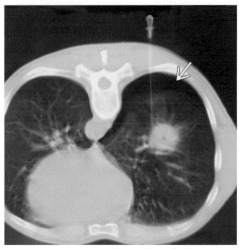

Pneumothorax (white arrow) occurred after initial needle biopsy attempt. Patient is prone.

- CT is helpful for masses with a pleural-based component, to avoid transgression of lung
- CT is convenient, sensitive way to check for post-procedure pneumothorax
- Larger the mass, easier it is to hit with a needle
- Closer mass is to chest wall, easier it is to hit
  - Closer mass is to diaphragm, more it moves
- If imaging appearance of nodule consistent with resectable carcinoma, it may be reasonable to proceed to surgical resection without biopsy
  - Some patients insist on biopsy prior to consenting for surgery

Patient Position and Prep
- Usually supine or prone
- Sometimes decubitus is best

Choice of Approach
- In general, shortest approach that goes through least amount of lung is best
- Ideal situation is when lesion can be approached without going through lung
- Things to avoid include subpleural blebs, bullae, large pulmonary artery or vein branches, liver and spleen

Monitoring
- Put patient on 2 liters O2 by nasal cannula
- Monitor pulse and oxygen saturation

Pathology Service
- Pathology service confirm specimen is adequate in amount and correctly processed
- Yield higher when pathology service present

CT-Guided Lung Biopsy
- Obtain images with 5 mm thick sections
- Place metallic BBs or other radiopaque marker on skin at level of lesion
- Repeat images with 4 cuts above and 4 cuts below level of lesion
- Choose your angle of approach

Lung Biopsy CT Guided

- Use CT scanner to measure distance from skin to lesion
- Prep, drape and give local anesthetic
- Place biopsy needle along planned path, but do not enter pleural space yet
- Repeat same set of 4 cuts above to 4 cuts below lesion to confirm that needle is along correct course
- Make sure needle stays in subcutaneous tissues, outside of chest during these manipulations
- Advance needle into lesion
- Remove stylet and apply 20 cm of suction to needle with a 20 cc syringe
- Gently give needle a 90° twist
- Obtain specimen and give to pathologist
- Wait while pathologist examines slides
- Check that patient is doing well
- If patient complains of shortness of breath, immediately re-scan

Post-Procedure
Things to Do
- After pathologist confirms specimen adequate, repeat CT of chest is obtained to confirm no pneumothorax
  o Usually 10 or 15 minutes after needle was removed
- Patient then sent to observation area and a follow-up portable chest x-ray is obtained in about 1 hour
- Patient should be accompanied by a responsible adult driver and given written discharge instructions

Common Problems & Complications
- Pneumothorax
- Hemoptysis
- Air embolism
- Pulmonary artery laceration
- Pericardial laceration with cardiac tamponade

Selected References
1. Dennie CJ et al: Transthoracic needle biopsy of lung: Results of early discharge in 506 outpatients. Radiology 219: 247-51, 2001
2. Cox J et al: Transthoracic needle aspiration biopsy: Variables that affect risk of pneumothorax. Radiology 212:165-8, 1999
3. Collings CL et al: Pneumothorax and dependent versus nondependent patient position after needle biopsy of lung. Radiology 210: 59-64, 1999

Lung Biopsy Fluoroscopic Guided

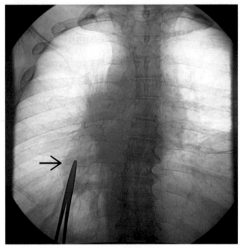

Hemostat tip (arrow) placed over posterior, left lung mass. Previous CT scan confirmed location and large size of mass. The patient is prone.

Key Facts
- Evaluate CT scan to determine best approach
- Consent for both lung biopsy and chest tube
- Adjust needle in soft tissues outside chest until course is correct
  - Then advance into lung mass
- Pathology service should be present

Pre-Procedure
Indications
- Lung mass

Contraindications
- No safe approach
  - E.g. surrounded by bullae
- INR over 1.4, especially with deep lesions
- Uncooperative patient

Consent
- Consent for both lung biopsy and possible chest tube
- It is better to have explained possible need for a chest tube in advance so that if needed will be ready

Getting Started
- Things to Check
  - Prior CT scan of chest
  - Someone in vicinity knows how to place chest tube
  - Tension pneumothoraces can happen suddenly
  - Reserve time in fluoroscopy suite
- Equipment List
  - 22-gauge, 9 cm long Franseen biopsy needle, works well
  - Many other types of needles can also be used
  - If 22-gauge unsuccessful, can try 20-gauge
  - Have chest tube available

Lung Biopsy Fluoroscopic Guided

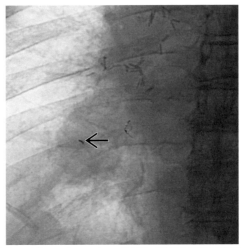

Needle hub (arrow) is superimposed over the tip so that it will travel in straight line. Note: Needle placed immediately above rib. Texture change felt when needle entered mass and needle tip location confirmed in AP, lateral and oblique views.

Procedure
Choice of Imaging Modality
- Large masses can often be biopsied with fluoroscopy, which is fastest method
- CT is helpful for masses with a pleural based component, so that transgression of lung can be avoided
- Larger mass, easier to hit with a needle
- Closer mass is to chest wall, easier to hit
- Closer mass is to diaphragm, more it will move with respiration and each breath hold
  - o Moving targets difficult to hit with needle
  - o All else being equal, go after lesion located more cephalad
- If imaging appearance of nodule consistent with resectable lung carcinoma, it may be reasonable to simply proceed to surgical resection without a biopsy
  - o Because even if biopsy negative for cancer, result may be considered indeterminate and surgery recommended
- Some patients will insist on a biopsy prior to consenting for surgery

Patient Position and Prep
- Usually supine or prone
- Sometimes decubitus is best

Choice of Approach
- In general, shortest approach that goes through least amount of lung is best
- Ideal situation is when lesion can be approached without going through lung so that there is no risk of pneumothorax
- Things to avoid include subpleural blebs, bullae, large pulmonary artery or vein branches, heart, liver and spleen

Monitoring
- Put patient on 2 L O_2 by nasal cannula

Lung Biopsy Fluoroscopic Guided

- Monitor pulse and oxygen saturation

Pathology Service
- Pathology service confirm specimen is adequate in amount and correctly processed
- Yield higher when pathology service present

Fluoroscopy-Guided Biopsy
- Angle image intensifier in bilateral oblique planes until optimal approach chosen
- Place needle along planned path, but do not enter pleural space yet
- Superimpose needle hub, tip and lesion
  o Ensures needle traveling in straight line parallel to x-ray beam
- Make sure needle stays in subcutaneous tissues outside of chest during these manipulations
- Advance needle into lesion
- Check orthogonal views to confirm needle in lesion
- Obtain specimen and give to pathologist
- If patient complains of shortness of breath, check fluoroscopy for evidence of pneumothorax

Post-Procedure

Things to Do
- After pathologist confirms specimen adequate, take a look with fluoroscopy to confirm no large pneumothorax present
- Seated, upright frontal chest x-ray in expiration and inspiration is obtained
- Do not send patient out of department until have checked chest x-ray
- Patient then sent to observation area and a follow-up portable chest x-ray is obtained in about 1 hour
- Patient should be accompanied by a responsible adult driver and given written discharge instructions

Common Problems and Complications

- False negative biopsy
- Pneumothorax
- Hemoptysis
  o Can lead to aspiration into contralateral lung
- Air embolism
- Pulmonary artery laceration
- Pericardial laceration with cardiac tamponade

Selected References
1. Dennie CJ et al: Transthoracic needle biopsy of the lung: Results of early discharge in 506 patients. Radiology 219: 247-51, 2001
2. Cox J et al: Transthoracic needle aspiration biopsy: Variables that affect risk of pneumothorax. Radiology 212:165-8, 1999
3. Collings CL et al: Pneumothorax and dependent versus nondependent patient position after needle biopsy of the lung. Radiology 210: 59-64, 1999

Thoracentesis

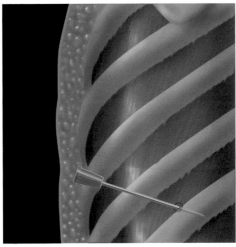

Needle for thoracentesis is placed over rib and into pleural space.

Key Facts
- Ultrasound (U/S) guidance increases success rate and safety of thoracentesis
- Obtain consent for thoracentesis and possible chest tube

Pre-Procedure
Indications
- Pleural effusion

Contraindications
- Uncorrectable bleeding diathesis

Getting Started
- Things to Check
  - Platelets, PTT, INR
  - Preprocedure chest x-ray (CXR)
    - If there really is an effusion
    - Location of effusion
    - Decubitus view helpful to show if free flowing
  - CT scan of chest if any
    - Provides much more information than CXR
  - Consent for thoracentesis and possible chest tube
  - Better to have explained possible need for chest tube in advance so if needed will be ready
- Equipment List
  - Thoracentesis kit
  - Blood gas syringe for pH with ice filled bag for transport to blood gas lab
  - Red top tube for chemistries including protein, glucose, LDH, amylase
  - Purple top tube for cell count
  - Blood culture bottles, aerobic and anaerobic
  - Sterile specimen container for Gram stain
    - Test tube like containers that come with thoracentesis kits are adequate

Thoracentesis

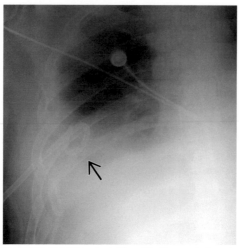

The diagnosis of acute empyema was confirmed by thoracentesis and a right-sided 16 French chest tube (arrow) was placed for thrombolysis and drainage of empyema.

- Otherwise, specimen can be put into a sterile urine specimen container
  o Sterile specimen (e.g. sterile urine type plastic) container for cytology
    - Try to obtain 20 or more cc for cytology
  o Have a chest tube, hemostat, Pleur-evac and related supplies available
  o Make sure that someone in vicinity knows how to put in a chest tube
    - Tension pneumothoraces are uncommon, but can happen suddenly
    - Also, if frank pus is obtained, chest tube can be placed at same setting

Procedure
Patient Position
- Sitting with legs over side of bed and a Mayo table-like stand in front of them to lean on
- An assistant should stand in front of patient

Procedure Steps
- Confirm all supplies are present before starting
- Administer 2 liters oxygen by nasal canula
- Open thoracentesis kit
  o Assemble three-way stopcock, drainage bag tubing and other supplies
- Identify entry site with U/S
- Give local anesthetic with a 25 to 30-gauge needle
- Make a skin nick for thoracentesis catheter
  o If don't make a skin nick, may damage catheter tip
  o Once tip damaged, it is unusable
  o Advance needle over rib to avoid neurovascular bundle which is located under rib
- Can make initial puncture with a smaller "finder" needle

Thoracentesis

o Obtaining pleural fluid confirms location
- Problem with small finder needles is that pleural fluid may be thick pus and not go thru small needle
  o Thick pus is rare, even with empyemas, can usually get some fluid with a 20-gauge needle
- Obtain a specimen for blood gas analysis
- Obtain specimen for other lab tests
- If adequate specimen obtained, put more in blood culture bottles as this increases yield

Post-Procedure
Things to Do
- Send specimens to laboratory
- Obtain post-procedure CXR
- Monitor patient
  o Patient remains in department until CXR confirmed negative

Common Problems & Complications
- Pneumothorax (PTx)
  o If get air in syringe, may be in lung and entry site too high
  o This is a warning sign that might have a pneumothorax
  o Obtain serial CXRs for small, asymptomatic PTx
  o Needle thoracostomy or chest tube used to treat larger, symptomatic PTx
  o For more information on chest tubes, please see chapter on chest tubes
- Laceration of intercostal artery, liver, spleen and heart
- Hemothorax
- Infection

Selected References
1. Gervais DA et al: US-guided thoracentesis: Requirement for postprocedure chest radiography in patients who receive mechanical ventilation versus patients who breathe spontaneously. Radiology 204:503-6, 1997
2. Aquino SL et al: Pleural exudates and transudates: Diagnosis with contrast-enhanced CT. Radiology 192:803-8, 1994
3. Harnsberger HR et al: Rapid, inexpensive real-time directed thoracentesis. Radiology 146:545-6, 1983

Shoulder Arthrogram

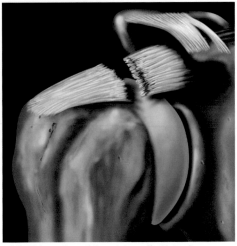

Full-thickness tear of the rotator cuff with tendinous gap.

Key Facts
- Shoulder arthrography involves injection of contrast into glenohumeral joint, obtaining x-rays and then CT or MRI images

Pre-Procedure
<u>Indications</u>
- Diagnosis of rotator cuff tears and glenoid labrum injuries
- Evaluation of shoulder instability and glenohumeral ligaments
- Evaluation of long head of biceps tendon attachment to labrum
- Loose body in shoulder joint
- Persistent symptoms after rotator cuff surgery
- Adhesive capsulitis of glenohumeral joint

<u>Contraindications</u>
- Infection of skin over joint
- Uncorrectable bleeding diathesis

<u>Getting Started</u>
- Things to Check
  - Bleeding history, platelets, PT, PTT, INR
  - Check location and pattern of symptoms
- Equipment List
  - 22-gauge spinal needle and connector tubing
  - Can use a myelogram kit as provides needle and connector tubing
  - Iodinated contrast e.g. Omnipaque 300 in a 5 cc syringe
  - Gadolinium and a 1 cc syringe

Procedure
<u>Patient Position</u>
- Supine with shoulder in neutral or externally rotated position

<u>Procedure Steps</u>
- Obtain scout views e.g. AP internal rotation (IR) and external rotation (ER)
  - For IR view, hands are pronated and for ER view, hands are supinated

Shoulder Arthrogram

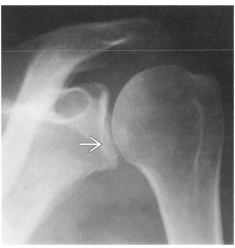

(Arrow) points to target level of glenohumeral joint for needle placement at junction of middle and lower thirds of the joint space.

- o For neutral view, palms are placed against legs
- Needle target is junction of middle and lower one third of curvilinear lucency that represents shoulder joint
  - o Needle should be placed along lateral/humeral side of joint line to avoid contact with glenoid labrum
- Use a "straight down" vertical approach to enter joint
  - o Helps avoid contact with glenoid labrum
  - o Allows use of fixed position fluoroscopy units
- Put target in center of field of view (FOV), magnify, and collimate
- Administer local anesthetic
- Superimpose hub over tip for straight line advancement
- Advance needle in increments, straight down into joint
- Confirm in joint with fluoroscopy and injection of 1 to 2 cc iodinated contrast
- When in joint, contrast will flow away from needle
  - o If contrast pools at needle tip, then not in joint

Double Contrast Arthrogram for Post-Arthrogram CT
- Iodinated contrast is first agent and air is second contrast agent
- Inject contrast along with 6 to 10 cc of air to obtain a double contrast arthrogram

MRI Arthrogram
- Draw up 15 cc sterile saline in a 20 cc syringe
- Use a 1 cc syringe to draw up 0.1 cc of gadolinium
- Add gadolinium to 20 cc syringe and remove bubbles
- Inject 8-12 cc into shoulder joint after needle location confirmed by injection of iodinated contrast

Anatomy
- Shoulder joint is also called glenohumeral joint
- Rotator cuff consists of supraspinatus, infraspinatus, teres minor and subscapularis muscles and their tendons
- Supraspinatus tendon is located along cephalad aspect of humeral head

Shoulder Arthrogram

- Supraspinatus tendon separates joint from subacromial-subdeltoid bursa
- A normal arthrogram will show contrast in glenohumeral joint, axillary recess, and subscapular recess
- A full-thickness tear of supraspinatus tendon allows contrast to pass from glenohumeral joint up into subacromial-subdeltoid bursa

Views
- Arm is moved thru range of motion to distribute contrast
- Obtain plain film postcontrast views while patient is supine in AP IR and AP ER projections
  - Also obtain an axillary view and "shoot through Y" lateral view
- For postcontrast MRI with shoulder in neutral position, obtain T1 coronal, T2 fat saturation (FS) coronal, T1 FS coronal, sagittal and axial
  - 3 or 4 mm thick images with 14 cm field of FOV
- Do not image in IR position, because causes angulation of supraspinatus tendon which makes it more difficult to interpret coronal images
- Also obtain T1 FS images in axial plane with shoulder in abduction and ER position
- Try to obtain CT or MRI images soon after injection, preferably within 60 minutes or less

Post-Procedure
Things to Do
- Observe patient for 15 minutes after CT or MRI and instruct to call if develops signs of infection

Common Problems & Complications
- Vasovagal episode e.g. in young, adult males
- Failure to enter joint e.g. with injection of subcoracoid bursa
- Fluid from therapeutic injections by referral service obscuring MRI findings
- Infection

Selected References
1. Lee SY et al: Horizontal component of partial-thickness tears of rotator cuff: Imaging characteristics and comparison of ABER view with oblique coronal view at MR arthrography-Initial results. Radiology 224: 470-6, 2002
2. Chung CB et al: MR Arthrography of the glenohumeral joint: A tailored approach. AJR 177:217-9, 2001
3. Roger B et al: Imaging findings in dominant shoulder of throwing athletes: comparison of radiography, arthrography, CT arthrography, and MR arthrography with arthroscopic correlation. AJR 172:1371-80, 1999

Chest Tube

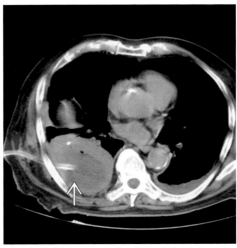

24 French chest tube (arrow) placed into right-sided empyema.

Key Facts
- Chest tubes are placed into pleural space with ultrasound and/or fluoroscopic guidance for treatment of pneumothorax, pleural effusion and empyema
  - CT guidance may also be used, especially for loculated collections

Pre-Procedure
Indications
- Symptomatic or large pneumothorax e.g. tension pneumothorax
- Symptomatic malignant pleural effusion
- Empyema

Contraindications
- Uncorrectable bleeding diathesis and infection at planned site of entry

Getting Started
- Things to Check
  - Bleeding history, platelets, PT, PTT, INR and respiratory status
  - Check previous imaging studies especially CT scan
    - Check location and amount of fluid
    - Check for signs of empyema or malignancy
    - Determine angle of approach and appropriate chest tube size
    - If collection contains air, then ultrasound unlikely to be helpful for entry and procedure should be done in CT
- Equipment List
  - 18-gauge (G) entry needle for Seldinger technique
  - 0.035" Amplatz, extra stiff, 75 cm long guidewire for Seldinger technique
  - Serial dilators from 5 French (Fr) to Fr size of chest tube to be placed
  - Hemostat and 3-0 monofilament nylon suture to secure tube
  - 2 inch or 3 inch silk tape to secure tube
  - Many companies make tubes from 9 to 16 Fr, suitable for chest drainage

Chest Tube

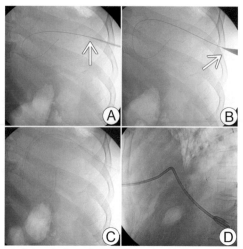

(A) Seldinger technique for large diameter chest tube placement with 9 French dilator & 0.038 extra stiff guidewire (arrow). (B) 22 French dilator (arrow) to further dilate tract. (C) 24 French chest tube placed in posterior costophrenic sulcus for drainage of pleural effusion. (D) 16 French chest tube with locking loop.

- o Cook company makes a Thal-Quik large diameter tube for placement with Seldinger technique
- o Comes in sizes 16-28 Fr and kit includes guidewire and dilators

Procedure

Patient Position
- Supine
- Ultrasound with fluoroscopy is preferred method of imaging guidance
- In general, helpful to enter as anterior as possible
- E.g. between mid-axillary line (MAL) and mid-clavicular line (MCL)
- Chest tubes placed posterior to MAL frequently become kinked
- At times a posterior approach is necessary for loculated collections

Determining Size of Tube
- Air collections, such as post thoracentesis or post biopsy pneumothoraces, can be drained with relatively small tubes such as 9-14 Fr
- In general a large bore tube e.g. at least 24 Fr is preferable for empyemas
  - o Medium size tubes e.g. 14 to 16 Fr can work well for treatment of empyema when fibrinolytics are administered
- When suspect empyema, drain as soon as possible because become increasingly septated and undrainable over time and may require surgery

Try to Minimize Pain During Chest Tube Placement
- Preemptive analgesia, such as intercostal nerve block and IV sedation, is more effective, than sedation after pain occurs
- Make sure have a good skin wheal and infiltrate down to periosteum
- Avoid letting tip of tube hit apical pleural surface, as this can be painful
- Secure tube well, because if tube falls out and needs to be replaced, second tube can be more painful
- Avoid excess separation of intercostal muscles with hemostat

Chest Tube

- o Excessively big hole in chest wall may increase fluid or air leakage
- Can inject local anesthetic into pleural cavity after draw off lab specimens
  - o Lidocaine is bacteriostatic and can change pleural fluid pH

Placement Technique
- Place 18 G needle in pleural space and confirm by aspiration of fluid or air
- Advance 0.035", Amplatz, extra stiff guidewire under fluoroscopic guidance
- Steer guidewire to desired location, e.g. posterior costophrenic angle for drainage of pleural effusion, this may require hockey-tip type catheter
- Dilate tract with serially increasing size dilators
- Place chest tube into desired location and confirm with fluoroscopy
- Secure tube to skin on medial and lateral sides of tube with 3-0 monofilament nylon suture
- Connect to collection system, e.g. Pleur-evac
- Tape chest tube and tubing securely
- Obtain baseline CXR

Post-Procedure
Things to Do
- Obtain daily, early morning portable CXR and follow tube output, check tube function, e.g. suction and water seal intact and tube tidals
- CT scans can be very helpful for clarification of CXR findings and to confirm adequate drainage
- Tube can be removed when drainage is complete based on clinical and imaging findings
- Analgesic medication immediately before removal, 4x4 gauze, Vaseline gauze, Betadine ointment, suture removal kit, Tegaderm/clear plastic adhesive dressing and silk tape are used for chest tube removal
- Order postprocedure portable CXR before remove tube, so that film will be obtained reasonably soon after tube removal

Common Problems & Complications
- Pain, infection and bleeding
- Kinking
- Occlusion by blood clot or empyema debris
- Air leak
- Subcutaneous emphysema
- Inadvertent dislodgement
- Disconnection of tubing can be minimized by taping all connections
- If collection bottle e.g. Pleur-evac tips over, then replace with new one
- Malposition, e.g. not in fluid collection is less likely with imaging guidance
- Pulmonary artery, cardiac injury, lung, liver, or spleen injury
- Winged scapula
- Horner's syndrome

Selected References
1. Parulekar W et al: Use of small-bore vs. large-bore chest tubes for treatment of malignant pleural effusions. Chest 120:19-25, 2001
2. Pien GW et al: Use of an implantable pleural catheter for trapped lung syndrome in patients with malignant pleural effusion. Chest 119:1641-6, 2001
3. Chang YC et al: Pneumothorax after small-bore catheter placement for malignant pleural effusions. AJR 166:1049-51, 1996

PocketRadiologist™
Interventional
Top 100 Procedures

ABDOMEN

Biliary Drainage

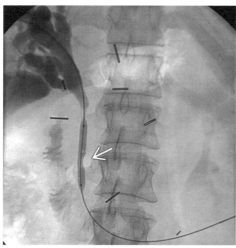

PTC shows biliary dilation due to malignancy of CBD, which was traversed with a glidewire. Exchange then made for extra stiff wire to facilitate balloon advancement. Note: Waist in balloon during angioplasty at site of obstruction (arrow). Now an internal-external catheter or metallic stent can be placed.

Key Facts
- Synonyms: Percutaneous biliary drainage (PBD)
- Percutaneous access to biliary system can be used for placement of drainage catheter, metal stent, stone removal, radiation brachytherapy, endoluminal biopsy or as a landmark for fluoroscopic biopsy

Pre-Procedure
Indications
- Most common indication is malignant biliary obstruction with unsuccessful attempt at ERCP (endoscopic retrograde cholangiopancreatography)
- Previous intestinal surgery which precludes ERCP
- Benign biliary obstruction with unsuccessful ERCP

Contraindications
- Uncorrectable bleeding diathesis
- Polycystic liver disease

Getting Started
- Things to Check
  - Bleeding history, platelets, PT, PTT, INR, creatinine and bilirubin
  - Check prior CT scan, ERCP, MRCP (magnetic resonance cholangiopancreatography) and related studies
  - Evaluation of an IV contrast enhanced CT scan is helpful for planning PBD
  - Administer antibiotics to all patients
- Equipment List
  - 21-gauge needle and 0.018" guidewire with coaxial dilator to upsize system
  - 0.035" angled tip regular and stiff type glidewires
  - 40 cm long, 5 French hockey-stick-tip catheter
  - 0.035", 145 cm long, Amplatz, extra stiff guidewire

Biliary Drainage

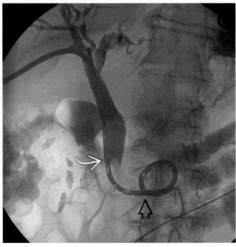

10 French internal-external biliary drainage catheter traverses malignant obstruction (curved arrow) of the common bile duct. Note: Catheter positioned so sideholes are proximal and distal to neoplasm. Distal loop (open arrow) locks catheter into duodenum.

Procedure
Patient Position
- Supine

Procedure Steps
- Perform PTC and obtain AP, RAO and LAO spot films
- Place 0.018" guidewire into a peripheral intrahepatic bile duct
- Use Seldinger technique to place a coaxial dilator, 0.035" guidewire and then a 5 French hockey-stick-tip catheter
- Advance hockey-stick catheter adjacent to site of obstruction and probe with a 0.035", angled-tip glidewire until wire crosses lesion
  - May need to use several different catheters and/or a stiff, 0.035", angled-tip glidewire to cross lesion
  - A torque device can be used to help steer guidewire
- If initially unable to cross lesion, can place an 8 French external drainage catheter and bring patient back in 2-7 days
  - With system now decompressed, may be able to cross lesion
- Once across lesion, advance guidewire into duodenum and then jejunum
- Follow guidewire with 5 French hockey-stick catheter
- Exchange glidewire for 0.035" Amplatz, extra stiff, 145 cm long guidewire
- Dilate tract to 8 French
- Place an 8 or 10 French internal-external biliary drainage (IE-BD) catheter
- Distal loop of IE-BD is formed in duodenum just beyond ampulla of Vater
- Loop is locked with a string which runs thru catheter
- Inject contrast to confirm sideholes are patent and are both proximal and distal to site of biliary obstruction
- Suture catheter to skin or adhesive device with 3-0 monofilament nylon

External Biliary Drain (E-BD)
- Connects to an external drainage bag which patient needs to drain several times each day

Biliary Drainage

- Electrolytes are lost in bile that is drained, and need to be replaced orally or intravenously e.g. with lactated Ringer's intravenous fluid
- External drains, while often necessary, are not a first choice method of drainage because of extra work and discomfort involved for patient associated with daily catheter care and loss of bile salts

<u>Internal-External Biliary Drain (IE-BD)</u>
- IE-BDs can only be placed when obstruction is traversed by a guidewire
- Catheter has an internal component and an external component
- Internal component consists of distal part of catheter with multiple sideholes both proximal and distal to site of obstruction and a locking loop for securing catheter in duodenum
- External component allows outward drainage of bile from patient
- External component maintains percutaneous access to biliary system which facilitates performance of subsequent procedures

<u>Metal Stent</u>
- Self-expanding metal stents can be placed across biliary obstructions

Post-Procedure
- Bed rest x 6 hours and continue antibiotics
- Flush forward only with 5-10 cc sterile saline q 8 hours for 1st week
  - More frequent flushing may be necessary if hemobilia is present
- Follow drain output, electrolytes, hemoglobin, white blood cell count and bilirubin
- Keep IE-BD catheter to external drainage for at least 5 days
  - Usually, may then cap off external port of IE-BD and allow patient to drain internally
- Replace electrolyte losses which can especially be significant with prolonged external drainage

Common Problems & Complications
- Pain
- Catheter occlusion, dislodgement and skin site infection
- Leakage of ascites around catheter
- Cholangitis and biliary sepsis
- Bleeding with perihepatic or intrahepatic hematoma or with hemobilia
- Metal stent erosion into duodenum with pain and/or bleeding

Selected References
1. Ernst O et al: Biliary Leaks: Treatment by means of percutaneous transhepatic biliary drainage. Radiology 211:345-8, 1999
2. Varghese JC et al: Role of MR cholangiopancreatography in patients with failed or inadequate ERCP. AJR 173:1527-33, 1999
3. Dinkel HP et al: Helical CT cholangiography for the detection and localization of bile duct leakage. AJR 173:613-7, 1999

Abscess Drainage

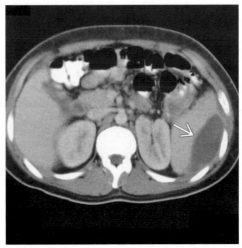

This perisplenic abscess (arrow) due to small bowel perforation was successfully treated with CT guided catheter drainage.

Key Facts
- Imaging-guided needle aspiration or percutaneous catheter drainage is an effective way to treat a majority of abdominal abscesses
- Imaging diagnosis of abscess can be challenging
  - Administration of additional contrast IV, oral, rectal or thru a urinary bladder catheter can be helpful to confirm diagnosis
- Typically needle aspiration alone is done for small collections
- Larger collections may require placement of a drainage catheter

Pre-Procedure
<u>Indications</u>
- Intraabdominal abscess
  - Common locations include subphrenic, perihepatic, perisplenic, paracolic gutter, iliopsoas, abdominal wall and pelvis
- To determine microorganism causing infection
- To decompress and drain pus so that antibiotics will be effective
<u>Contraindications</u>
- No safe route for drainage e.g. due to lesion being surrounded by bowel
- Uncorrectable bleeding diathesis
<u>Getting Started</u>
- Things to Check
  - Carefully review CT scan to confirm an abscess is actually present
  - Abscesses can be difficult to detect on a CT scan
  - Non-opacified bowel is not uncommonly mistaken for an abscess
  - When in doubt, try to obtain better images
    - Can give IV contrast and obtain delayed images so that contrast fills urinary bladder to distinguish it from fluid in pouch of Douglas
    - Can put contrast into urinary bladder thru a Foley catheter
    - Consider giving more oral contrast
    - Consider rectal contrast

Abscess Drainage

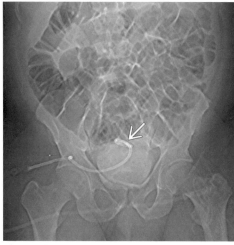

Transgluteal approach drainage catheter (arrow) placed within a pelvic abscess.

- o Plan approach to lesion
- o In general, shortest route that does not traverse any important structure is preferred
- o Check bleeding history, platelets, PT, PTT, INR
- o Get all supplies ready before starting procedure
- o Confirm that patient has good IV access and is receiving antibiotics
- • Equipment List
  - o An 18-gauge needle is usually used for puncture of abscesses
    - ▪ Can be used to aspirate fluid and for placement of drains with Seldinger technique
  - o Amplatz, extra stiff, 0.035" diameter, 75 cm long guidewire
  - o Dilators e.g. 5, 7, 9, and 11 French
  - o Catheters designed for abscess drainage including "all purpose drains"
    - ▪ Catheters have a locking mechanism to prevent dislodgement
    - ▪ These catheters have larger side holes than nephrostomy catheters
    - ▪ 10 Fr is a useful size for most moderate to large size abscesses

Things to Avoid
- • Bowel, especially colon
- • Pleural space
- • Large blood vessels
- • Spleen
- • Intraabdominal hematomas that are unlikely to be infected

Procedure
Patient Position
- • Supine or prone
Procedure Steps
- • CT is most common method of imaging guidance for abscess drainage
  - o Ultrasound and fluoroscopy are helpful for some lesions
- • Obtain CT scan with 8-10 mm thick images

Abscess Drainage

- Place some form of radiopaque marker on patient's skin at level of lesion
- Repeat CT scan with 4 images above and 4 images below lesion
- Use markers as a guide to where to place needle thru skin
- Advance 18-gauge needle into lesion
- Aspirate with a syringe and put specimen in a sterile container
  - Send to laboratory for Gram stain and culture
- Abscesses too small for catheter placement can be irrigated thru a needle with sterile saline
- For larger abscesses, place a guidewire into lesion
- Dilate tract to desired size
- Advance drainage tube over Amplatz guide wire and into abscess
- Advance metal stiffener up to abscess margin, but no further
- Will experience loss of resistance when plastic part of drainage tube passes into abscess
- Fix position of metal stiffener, and advance drainage tube into abscess
- Repeat CT images to confirm catheter is in correct location
- Consider irrigating abscess
- Sew catheter to patient's skin or an adhesive device on skin
- Tape catheter securely with mesentery-style taping

Post-Procedure
Things to Do
- Bed rest x 6 hours
- Check blood pressure, pulse and inquire regarding abdominal pain q 15 min x 1, q 30 min x 1, q 1 hour x 5 hours
  - Record catheter output on graphics sheet q shift
  - Flush catheter with 10 cc sterile, normal saline q 8 hours
- Follow catheter output, WBC (white blood cell count), fever and pain
- Persistent fever and leukocytosis after 1 to 2 days often indicates undrained pus and a repeat CT scan should be obtained
- Signs of improvement include normalization of WBC count, afebrile, return of hemodynamic stability and resolution of abscess on CT scan

Common Problems & Complications
- Inadequate drainage due to loculated collection or fistula
- Abscesses unable to be drained percutaneously often require open surgery
- Bleeding
- Puncture of bowel
- Pneumothorax and empyema if diaphragm is traversed
- Catheter dislodgement
- Bacteremia and septic shock
- Inadvertent dislodgement of tube

Selected References
1. Catalano OA et al: Efficacy of percutaneous abscess drainage with vancomycin-resistant enterococci. AJR 175:533-6, 2000
2. Rajak CL et al: Percutaneous treatment of liver abscess: Needle aspiration versus catheter drainage. AJR 170:1035-9, 1998
3. D'Agostine HB et al: Influence of the stopcock on the efficiency of percutaneous drainage catheters: Laboratory evaluation. AJR 159:407-9, 1992

Gastrostomy

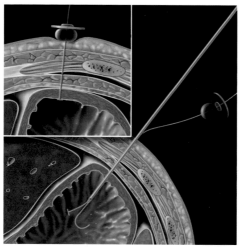

Placement of T-fasteners. Needle containing fastener placed through abdominal wall and anterior wall of stomach, air aspirated and contrast injected. Wire pushes fastener into stomach. Fastener pulled up to hold stomach wall against anterior abdominal wall (insert).

Key Facts
- Procedure synonyms: G-tube placement, PEG (refers to endoscopic placement, request for PEG even if tube to be placed by radiology)
- Procedure definition: Placement of tube through anterior abdominal wall into the stomach
- Clinical setting: Unable to take oral feedings; gastric decompression
- Most feared complications: Puncturing structures in close proximity (liver, bowel); tube dislodged into peritoneal cavity leading to peritonitis

Pre-Procedure
Indications
- Long-term nutritional support
  - Impairing swallowing–esophageal obstruction, CNS disease
- Gastric decompression
Absolute Contraindications
- Lack of safe access into stomach, uncorrectable coagulopathy, ventriculoperitoneal shunt
Relative Contraindications
- Previous gastric surgery, gastric varices, gastric cancer, peritoneal carcinomatosis may require CT for placement
- Ascites requires gastropexy and paracentesis
- Severe gastroesophageal reflux – gastrojejunal tube placement
Getting Started
- Things to Check
  - Previous imaging, CT scans of abdomen (position of colon)
  - Contrast via NG tube night prior, opacify colon, or contrast enema at procedure if colon not visible fluoroscopically
  - NG tube in place to inflate stomach
  - Patient NPO 12 hours prior to procedure
- Equipment List

Gastrostomy

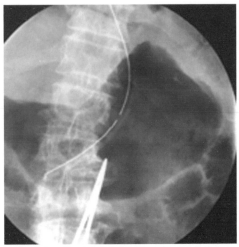

Selecting area for gastrostomy tube placement. Stomach inflated with air. Clamp marks puncture site, over the mid-body of stomach. NG in place.

- Ultrasound to mark position of left lobe of liver
- T-fasteners, used to perform gastropexy
- Wire – LT, Amplatz super stiff
- Teflon dilators to size of gastrostomy tube
- Gastrostomy tube
  - Catheters 10-20 Fr, multiple side holes
  - Retention devices – Cope loop or balloon
- Glucagon 1 mg, lidocaine, sedation

Procedure
Patient Position/Location
- Supine with fluoroscopy, ultrasound used to mark left lobe of liver

Equipment Preparation
- Load T-fasteners into needle

Procedure Steps
- Prep anterior abdominal wall in region of stomach
- IV Glucagon to decrease peristalsis
- Insufflate stomach via NG tube, **monitor** with fluoroscopy, be careful not to over distend
- Select site for puncture, subcostal, left of midline, anesthetize skin
- Insert needle containing T-fastener into stomach under fluoroscopy – visualize stomach indention, aspiration of air when stomach entered, contrast injected to confirm position
- Wire through needle dislodges T-fastener, needle/wire removed, fastener withdrawn at skin, tacks anterior wall of stomach to abdominal wall
- T-fasteners, optimally 3 in a triangular configuration, 1 better than none, 2 better than 1
- T-fasteners placed, skin incision in center of fasteners, tissues dissected
- Needle through incision into stomach, wire placed, tract dilated
- Catheter placed and contrast injected to confirm proper positioning

Gastrostomy

<u>Alternative Procedures/Therapies</u>
- Surgical
  - o Surgical gastrostomy not widely performed - cost and complications
- Endoscopic placement
  - o Endoscope must be positioned in stomach, transilluminate abdominal wall
  - o Difficult in post-operative stomach

Post-Procedure
<u>Things to Do</u>
- No feeding until next day, no evidence of peritonitis
- Increase feedings slowly to avoid over-distension of stomach
- T-fasteners cut 10-14 days post procedure
- G tube should be replaced on regular basis, q 6 months
<u>Things to Avoid</u>
- Pills through gastrostomy
- Kinking, dislodgement of tube

Common Problems & Complications
<u>Problems</u>
- No space between liver, costal margin, bowel
  - o CT guidance, overnight rectal tube decompress colon
  - o Post-op stomach particularly a problem
- NG tube can not be placed
  - o Place 5-Fr catheter under fluoroscopic guidance
- T-fasteners not used, difficulty in dilating track
  - o Stomach pushed away by dilators
  - o Wire may prolapse between stomach and abdominal wall
  - o If not recognized tube may be placed into peritoneum
<u>Complications</u>
- Severe
  - o Peritonitis
  - o Hemorrhage
  - o Leakage
- Other complications
  - o Aspiration pneumonia
  - o Superficial skin infection
  - o Tube malfunction, tube dislodgement

Selected References
1. Ho SG et al: Radiological percutaneous gastrostomy. Clin Radiol 56:902-10, 2001
2. Giuliano AW et al: Fluoroscopically guided percutaneous placement of large-bore gastrostomy and gastrojejunostomy tubes: Review of 109 Cases. JVIR 11: 239-46, 2000
3. Ryan JM et al: Percutaneous gastrostomy with T-fastener gastropexy: Results of 316 consecutive procedures. Radiology 203:496-500, 1997

Gastrojejunostomy

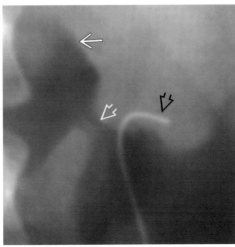

Using directional catheter to negotiate through the pylorus and duodenum prior to gastrojejunal tube placement. (White arrow) duodenal bulb, (white open arrow) pylorus, (black open arrow) directional catheter

Key Facts
- Procedure synonyms: GJ-tube placement
- Procedure definition: Placement of tube via stomach with tip of tube in proximal jejunum
- Clinical setting: Unable to take oral feedings and with gastroesophageal reflux
- Most feared complications: Puncturing structures in close proximity (liver, bowel)

Pre-Procedure
Indications
- Long-term nutritional support
  - Impaired swallowing–esophageal obstruction, CNS disease, and
  - Poor gastric emptying and/or gastroesophageal reflux
Absolute Contraindications
- Lack of safe access into stomach, uncorrectable coagulopathy, ventriculoperitoneal shunt
Relative Contraindications
- Previous gastric surgery, gastric varices, gastric cancer, peritoneal carcinomatosis may require CT for placement
- Ascites requires gastropexy and paracentesis
Getting Started
- Things to Check
  - Previous imaging, CT scans of abdomen (position of colon)
  - Contrast via NG tube night prior, opacify colon, or contrast enema at procedure if colon not visible fluoroscopically
  - NG tube in place to inflate stomach
  - Patient NPO 12 hours prior to procedure
- Equipment List
  - Ultrasound to mark position of left lobe of liver

Gastrojejunostomy

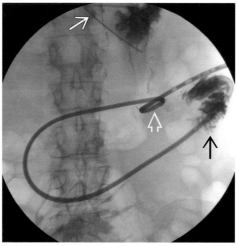

Placement of gastrojejunostomy tube. (White arrow) indicates NG tube. (Open arrow) demonstrates retention loop. (Black arrow) indicates tip of catheter in the proximal jejunum.

- o T-fasteners, used to perform gastropexy
- o Wires – LT wire standard length, Terumo hydrophilic wire exchange length, Amplatz super stiff wire exchange length
- o Directional catheters-Kumpe, Cobra, headhunter shapes
- o Teflon dilators to size of gastrojejunostomy tube
- o Gastrojejunostomy tube
  - 10-24 Fr, multiple side holes
  - Stomach retention devices – Cope loop, Mallecot, or balloon
- o Glucagon 1 mg (try to avoid, decreases motility which may be needed for the jejunal catheterization), Reglan 10 mg, lidocaine, sedation

Procedure
Patient Position/Location
- Supine with fluoroscopy, ultrasound used to mark left lobe of liver

Equipment Preparation
- Load T-fasteners into needle

Procedure Steps
- Preliminary steps through the insertion of the T-fasteners is described in gastrostomy chapter
- Avoid IV Glucagon if possible
- Needle through incision into stomach, **very important to direct needle towards the pylorus**
- Wire placed through the pylorus, if wire does not pass pylorus, then needle exchanged for directional catheter and attempts made to pass pylorus with directional catheter and hydrophilic wire
- If difficulty in passing pylorus, place 6-7 French angiographic sheath, allows easier catheter manipulation and injection of contrast to help visualize the duodenal bulb
- When wire and catheter positioned in proximal jejunum, exchange wire for a stiff wire

Gastrojejunostomy

- Place peel-away sheath, particularly for large bore catheters
- Place catheter with tip in proximal jejunum distal to ligament of Treitz
- Deploy retention device in stomach

Alternative Procedures/Therapies
- Surgical
  - o Surgical jejunostomy
- Endoscopic placement
  - o Endoscope must be positioned in stomach, transilluminate abdominal wall
  - o Difficult in post-operative stomach

Post-Procedure
Things to Do
- May feed immediately, liberal irrigation after each use
- T-fasteners cut 10-14 days post procedure
- Routine change of tube q 6 months

Things to Avoid
- Pills through gastrojejunostomy tube

Common Problems & Complications
Problems
- Difficulty negotiating into duodenum
  - o Contrast not moving through stomach and duodenum; Reglan 10 mg IV may be helpful in stimulating bowel motility
  - o Terumo wire may pass more easily than standard wires
  - o Cannot access duodenum, place G-tube, convert to GJ later
- T-fasteners crucial for tube placement success
- Patient requiring gastric decompression as well as feeding
  - o Double lumen gastrojejunostomy tube

Complications
- Severe
  - o Peritonitis
  - o Hemorrhage
  - o Leakage
- Other complications
  - o Superficial skin infection
  - o Tube malfunction, dislocation

Selected References
1. Giuliano AW et al: Fluoroscopically guided percutaneous placement of large-bore gastrostomy and gastrojejunostomy tubes: review of 109 cases. JVIR 11: 239-46, 2000
2. Dewald CL et al: Percutaneous gastrostomy and gastrojejunostomy with gastropexy: experience in 701 procedures. Radiology 211: 651-6, 1999
3. Bell SD et al: Percutaneous gastrostomy and gastrojejunostomy: additional experience in 519 procedures. Radiology 194:817-20, 1995

Liver Biopsy

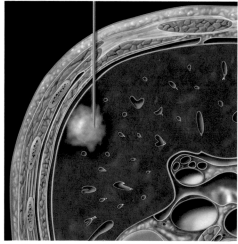

Needle path for biopsy is chosen such that some normal liver tissue is interposed between lesion and liver capsule. This helps to decrease risk of hemoperitoneum.

Key Facts
- Fine needle aspiration (FNA) of liver can be done with CT or ultrasound
- Smaller, deeper lesions, near dome are more difficult
- Yield is increased when pathology service is present at biopsy

Pre-Procedure
Indications
- Liver mass suspected of being malignant
- Hepatitis C
- Progressive diffuse liver disease
- Liver transplantation protocol

Contraindications
- Relative contraindications include suspected hemangioma and ascites

Getting Started
- Things to Check
  - o Check bleeding history, INR, PTT, platelets
  - o Stop aspirin for one week when cardiac status will tolerate
  - o Review previous ultrasound and CT
    - Check for intervening colon or large pleural effusion that extends around liver
  - o No solid foods for 8 hours prior to procedure
    - No liquids for 4 hours pre-procedure
  - o Yield is increased when pathology service is present at biopsy to evaluate and process specimens
- Equipment List
  - o 22-gauge, 9 cm long Franseen biopsy needle works well
    - 22-gauge is good size to start with for FNA
  - o If unsuccessful, can try 20-gauge
  - o Shorter needles bend less and are easier to steer
  - o Use shortest possible needle
  - o For lymphomas, a relatively large specimen is needed

Liver Biopsy

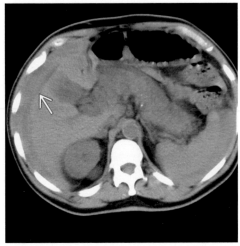

Massive hemoperitoneum following liver biopsy. Note: Layered appearance of blood with dense areas of clotted blood (arrow). The bleeding extended around the spleen and into the pelvis.

- ▪ Should discuss with pathologist
- o Core biopsy needle sizes vary from 14 to 18-gauge

Procedure

Patient Position
- Supine

Choice of Entry Site
- Try to interpose some normal-appearing liver between liver margin and lesion along needle tract
  - o Helps to prevent bleeding
  - o Especially for biopsy of possible hemangioma

Things to Avoid
- Large vessels such as IVC and portal vein
- Gallbladder
- Pleural space and lung
- Colon

Choice of Imaging Guidance for FNA
- Benefits of CT include increased visibility of most lesions, increased ability to check for post-procedure bleeding or pneumothorax, and usually technically less difficult than ultrasound
- Benefits of ultrasound include faster, more choices of route, easier for angulated approaches, real time visualization of needle, and usually more readily available for scheduling purposes than CT

Procedure Steps
- Measure lesion depth from skin surface and choose needle length
- For CT-guided biopsy, place metallic markers on skin in region of planned skin entry
- Things to avoid include lung, gallbladder, and large blood vessels
  - o Rarely, a transpulmonic approach may be necessary
- Be generous with local anesthetic

Liver Biopsy

- Place biopsy needle into lesion
- Confirm in lesion with ultrasound or CT
  - Obtain image of needle within lesion
- Apply 10 to 20 cm negative suction on syringe and make a single 180 degree twisting motion with needle
- Do not make excessive motions with needle as this just leads to bleeding which degrades specimen
- Specimen is given to pathology service
  - FNA specimens are placed onto slides
  - Core biopsy specimens are placed in formalin

Post-Procedure
Things to Do
- Bed rest x 5 hours for FNA
- NPO for 4 hours
- Check blood pressure, pulse and inquire regarding abdominal pain q 15 min x 2, q 30 min x 2, q 1 hour x 4
- Notify physician of any changes

Common Problems & Complications
- Bleeding
  - If suspect, obtain CT scan
  - Surgery or angioembolization may be necessary
- Mild persistent pain
  - Small amount of bleeding may irritate liver capsule
- Biliary colic due to hemobilia or gallbladder puncture with needle
- Pneumothorax
- Infection

Selected References
1. Plecha DM et al: Liver Biopsy: Effects of biopsy needle caliber on bleeding and tissue recovery. Radiology 204: 101-4, 1997
2. Little AF et al: Image-guided percutaneous hepatic biopsy: Effect of ascites on the complication rate. Radiology 199:79-83, 1996
3. Baker ME: What is the most cost-effective imaging workup for hepatic hemangiomas, and is it safe to obtain a biopsy of such a suspected hemangioma? AJR 163:1261, 1994

Pancreas Biopsy

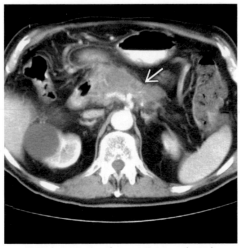

Typical appearance of pancreatic cancer (arrow).

Key Facts
- CT guidance is typically used for biopsy of pancreas
- Yield is increased when pathology service is present at biopsy

Pre-Procedure
Indications
- Pancreatic mass
  - Pancreatic adenocarcinoma is most common reason for biopsy
- Differentiation of chronic pancreatitis from pancreatic carcinoma
- Differentiation of pancreatic pseudocysts from cystic tumors
- To confirm suspected metastatic disease in a patient with a known malignancy elsewhere such as lung carcinoma
- Pancreatic and peripancreatic fluid collections are sometimes aspirated in setting of pancreatitis to check if fluid collection is infected
- Evaluation of pancreas transplant for rejection

Contraindications
- Uncooperative patient
- Uncorrectable bleeding diathesis
- Pseudoaneurysm due to pancreatitis

Getting Started
- Things to Check
  - Check bleeding history, INR, PTT, platelets
  - NPO status at least 6 hours prior to procedure is important
    - Stomach is often traversed with a needle during this procedure
    - Small bowel and colon are sometimes traversed
  - Review previous ultrasound and CT to confirm lesion and plan approach
    - IV contrast helps to delineate pancreatic lesions
    - Check for tumor in other locations such as liver which may be preferable site to biopsy
    - Check for intervening colon, stomach and normal pancreatic tissue

Pancreas Biopsy

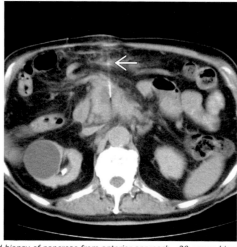

CT-guided biopsy of pancreas from anterior approach. 20-gauge biopsy (arrow).

- o Call pathology service in advance to confirm available
- Equipment
  - o Pancreatic biopsy is typically done with a 20-gauge biopsy needle
  - o Sometimes an 18-gauge needle is required
  - o Use shortest possible needle as these bend less and are easier to steer

Things to Avoid
- A dilated pancreatic duct
- Normal pancreas should be avoided when possible
- It is sometimes necessary to traverse some normal pancreatic tissue
- Try to minimize, as it seems that it is normal part of pancreas that is more likely to develop pancreatitis if traversed by needle
  - o For example, a needle may cause thrombus formation in pancreatic duct or injury to pancreatic duct
- Spleen should be avoided because of risk of bleeding
- It is usually safe to go thru bowel
- Given a choice, it is better to traverse small bowel rather than large bowel
- Stomach often needs to be traversed

Procedure
Patient Position
- Supine

Choice of Imaging Guidance
- Fine needle aspiration of pancreas can be done with CT or ultrasound
- Benefits of CT include increased visibility of most lesions, increased ability to check for post-procedure bleeding, and usually technically less difficult
- Benefits of ultrasound include faster, more choices of route, easier for angulated approaches, real time visualization of needle, and usually more readily available for scheduling purposes than CT
- Downside to CT is a lack of real time guidance
- Downside of ultrasound is usually only can identify relatively large lesions and often has poor visualization of pancreas due to bowel gas

Pancreas Biopsy

- If patient has an indwelling internal-external biliary drain and a large surrounding mass in pancreatic head, then can biopsy with fluoroscopy

Procedure Steps
- Measure lesion depth from skin surface and choose needle length
- For CT-guided biopsy, place metallic markers on skin in region of planned skin entry
- Be generous with local anesthetic
- Obtain 5 mm thick axial images thru pancreas
- Pass needle down to lesion
  - Obtain image of needle within lesion
- Apply 10 cm of negative suction to syringe and make a single 180 degree twisting motion with needle to obtain a specimen
- Do not make excessive motions with needle as this just leads to bleeding which degrades specimen
- Specimen is given to pathology service
  - FNA specimens are placed onto slides
  - Core biopsy specimens are usually placed in formalin
  - Fluid from pancreatic cysts can be sent for Gram stain, culture and amylase evaluation
  - Pathology service may also recommend additional tests such as evaluation for tumor markers like carcinoembryonic antigen (CEA)
- Make additional passes as necessary
- Obtain a post procedure CT scan to check for hemorrhage

Post-Procedure

Things to Do
- Bed rest and NPO x 4 hours
- Check blood pressure, pulse and inquire regarding abdominal pain q 15 min x 2, q 30 min x 2, q 1 hour x 3

Common Problems & Complications
- False negative biopsy result
- Bleeding
- Pain
- Injury to pancreatic or common bile duct
- Pancreatitis
  - Can be severe
- Pancreatic duct injury
- Ileus secondary to intestinal spasm after needle trauma
- Infection
  - Increased risk with colon traversal with a large needle en route to large cystic lesion in immunocompromised patient
- Tumor spread along needle tract

Selected References
1. Gupta S et al: Masses in or around the pancreatic head: CT-guided coaxial fine-needle aspiration biopsy with a posterior transcaval approach. Radiology 222:63-9, 2002
2. Balen FG et al: Biopsy of inoperable pancreatic tumors does not adversely influence patient survival time. Radiology 193:753-5, 1994
3. Brandt KR et al: CT - and US-guided biopsy of the pancreas. Radiology 187:99-104, 1993

Percutaneous Cholecystostomy

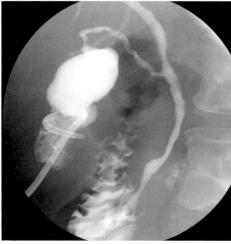

Acute cholecystitis. Cholecystosomy was placed with Seldinger technique as well as ultrasound and fluoroscopic guidance. 3 weeks later in asymptomatic patient, this followup cholangiogram shows patent ductal system. Tube removed after tractogram.

Key Facts
- Percutaneous cholecystostomy is placement of a drainage catheter into gallbladder (GB)
- Typical patient has acute cholecystitis or sepsis of unknown origin and is too ill due to comorbidities to undergo conventional surgery
- Use ultrasound whenever possible

Pre-Procedure
<u>Indications</u>
- Acute cholecystitis in patients too ill to undergo conventional surgery
- Sepsis of unknown origin with negative workup other than abnormal gallbladder ultrasound

<u>Contraindications</u>
- Uncorrectable bleeding diathesis

<u>Getting Started</u>
- Things to Check
  - Previous abdominal CT and ultrasound
    - Confirm GB abnormal, e.g. dilated with thick wall
    - For shrunken cirrhotic liver, ectopic gallbladder, and colon anterior to liver
    - For signs of perforation and bilomas which may require additional drainage catheter
    - Choose a transhepatic route to GB which avoids large vessels in liver
  - Check INR, PTT, and platelets
- Equipment List
  - Ultrasound is very helpful
    - Typically a curved 2 to 3.5 MHz transducer
  - In some large patients, gallbladder not visible with ultrasound

Percutaneous Cholecystostomy

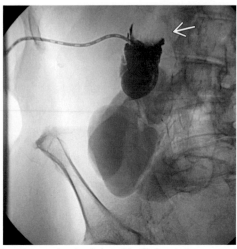

Stone in GB neck caused acute cholecystitis. Cholecystostomy was placed. Not a surgical candidate due to end stage COPD. Cholangiogram obtained 1 week after catheter placed shows large stone (arrow) obstructing GB neck. 4 weeks later, stone moved away from GB neck & contrast flowed into bile duct & duodenum.

- ▪ Procedure can be done with CT
  - o Fluoroscopy should also be used whenever possible
  - o It is preferable, when patient is able to be transported, to do procedure in interventional radiology (IR) department rather than at patient's bedside
    - ▪ Makes procedure easier because more equipment available
  - o Use an 18-gauge needle
    - ▪ Using a micropuncture needle adds steps and increases risk of losing access
  - o 0.035" guidewire with 3 mm J-type tip
  - o 8 French locking loop catheter with large sideholes

Procedure
Patient Position/Location
- • Supine
Procedure Steps
- • If procedure to be done portable, make a list of all things will need
  - o Bring an assistant to help with procedure
  - o It happens all too often that some piece of equipment is forgotten and someone needs to bring it from IR suite to ICU
- • Evaluate GB with ultrasound
- • Make a small nick in skin with # 11 scalpel
  - o Spread nick superficially with hemostat
- • Use ultrasound to guide 18-gauge needle into GB
  - o Will often see bile flow out of needle
- • Thread guidewire into gallbladder
  - o Try to see guidewire in gallbladder with ultrasound
- • Dilate tract to 8 French
- • Place 8 French drainage catheter

Percutaneous Cholecystostomy

- Rarely, bile will be quite thick and require catheter larger than 8 French
- Make sure to activate locking mechanism of catheter
- Suture catheter to skin with 3-0 monofilament nylon
  - Tape drainage tube securely to skin using silk tape and a mesentery technique
- Attach drainage tube to a gravity collection bag
  - If available, a closed system with a suction bulb-like effect is convenient because does not require dependent positioning
- Send bile for Gram stain, culture and cell count

Removal of a Percutaneous Cholecystostomy
- Tube can be removed after symptoms have resolved and a cholecystostogram shows cystic and common bile duct are patent
- Usually takes 2 to 4 weeks for tract of tube to mature so that bile will not leak when tube removed
- Remove tube over guidewire and inject tract
  - If tract leaks, place a new tube into GB
  - Wait another 1 to 2 weeks to allow more time for tract maturation
- Some patients will have improvement in clinical condition and be able to undergo surgical removal of GB

Alternative Procedures
- Surgical cholecystostomy
- Laparoscopic or open cholecystostomy

Post-Procedure

Things to Do
- Record drain output q shift
- Sudden decreased output suggests GB obstruction resolved, tube occluded or pulled out of GB
- Need to carefully examine catheter
  - Remove dressing to make sure catheter not pulled out and hiding under dressing
- Large volume outputs can cause electrolyte depletion
  - These need to be replaced

Common Problems & Complications
- Catheter dislodgement
  - CT scan for biloma
  - Follow patient closely
  - Some patients will do well and not need further intervention
  - Others will need cholecystostomy to be replaced, especially if has only been in less than 1 to 2 weeks
- Bile leak
- Bile peritonitis
- Bleeding
  - Bleeding may be due to injury of hepatic artery or vein, or portal vein
  - Severe bleeding may require transcatheter embolization or surgery

Selected References
1. England RE et al: Percutaneous cholecystostomy: Who responds? AJR 168:1247-51, 1997
2. Boland GW et al: Percutaneous cholecystostomy in critically ill patients: Early response and final outcome in 82 patients. AJR 163:339-42, 1994
3. Boland GW et al: Percutaneous cholecystostomy for acute acalculous cholecystitis in a critically ill patient (clinical conference). AJR 160:871-2, 1993

Transgluteal Abcess Drainage

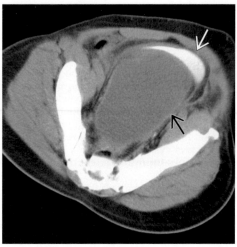

Large pelvis abscess (black arrow) mimics appearance of urinary bladder. Intravenous contrast given to opacify bladder (white arrow) was helpful to distinguish bladder from abscess. Subsequently a drainage catheter was placed with a transgluteal approach.

Key Facts
- Imaging diagnosis of deep pelvis abscess can be challenging
  - Administration of additional contrast IV, oral, rectal or thru urinary bladder catheter can be helpful to confirm diagnosis
- Needle is placed caudal to piriformis muscle and adjacent to sacrum

Pre-Procedure
Indications
- Pelvis abscess in pouch of Douglas
- An anterior approach to deep pelvis abscesses is often precluded by intervening bowel, bladder and blood vessels

Contraindications
- No safe route for drainage, e.g. due to rectum being distended with air
  - Decompression with a rectal tube and/or injection of saline into perirectal space may facilitate a safe path for needle

Getting Started
- Things to Check
  - Carefully review CT scan to confirm an abscess is actually present
  - Abscesses can be difficult to detect on a CT scan
  - Non-opacified bowel is not uncommonly mistaken for an abscess
  - When in doubt, try to obtain better images
    - Can give IV contrast and obtain delayed images so that contrast fills urinary bladder to distinguish it from fluid in pouch of Douglas
    - This method can be very helpful
    - Can put contrast into urinary bladder thru a Foley catheter
    - Consider giving more oral contrast or giving rectal contrast
  - Check bleeding history, platelets, PT, PTT, INR
  - Plan approach to lesion
    - Alternative routes include transrectal and transvaginal

Transgluteal Abcess Drainage

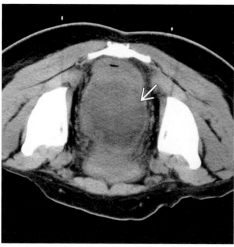

Large pelvic abscess (arrow). Note: Patient is prone, skin is visible on image, and metallic markers are placed on skin to denote level. Opacification of rectum with oral or rectal contrast and of urinary bladder with IV contrast can be very helpful.

- o Sacrospinous ligament extends from sacrum to ischial spine and separates greater and lesser sciatic foramina
- o Piriformis muscle is a useful landmark as sciatic nerve typically passes anterior to it and then exits pelvis along middle to lateral, inferior margin of muscle
- o Therefore try to place needle for drainage caudal to piriformis muscle and adjacent to sacrum and coccyx
- o Angled approach with needle directed slightly cephalad can be helpful
- o Superior gluteal nerves and arteries pass above piriformis muscle
- o Superior gluteal artery is largest branch of internal iliac artery
- o Inferior gluteal nerves pass below piriformis muscle
- Equipment List
  - o An 18-gauge needle is usually used for puncture of abscesses
  - o Amplatz, extra stiff, 0.035" diameter, 75 cm long guidewire
  - o Dilators e.g. 5, 7, 9, and 11 French
  - o Catheters designed for abscess drainage including "all purpose drains"
    - ▪ Catheters have a locking mechanism to prevent dislodgement
    - ▪ These catheters have larger sideholes than nephrostomy catheters
    - ▪ 8 to 12 French are useful sizes for most pelvis abscesses

Things to Avoid
- Rectum
- Sciatic nerve
- Large blood vessels

Procedure
Patient Position
- Prone
  - o Sometimes, slight elevation of one side towards a decubitus position will facilitate a clear path for needle

Transgluteal Abcess Drainage

Procedure Steps
- Obtain CT scan with 5-8 mm thick images
- Place some form of radiopaque marker on patient's skin at level of lesion
- Repeat CT scan with 4 images above and 4 images below lesion
- Use markers as a guide to where to place needle thru skin
- Drainage catheter can be placed with trocar or Seldinger technique
- A small diameter "finder" needle is initially placed to guide the trocar
- For Seldinger technique an 18-gauge needle is first placed into lesion
- Aspirate with a syringe and put specimen in a sterile container
- Small abscesses can be aspirated with needle
  - However, aspiration alone increases risk of recurrent abscess
- For larger abscesses, a guidewire is placed into lesion and tract is dilated
- Advance drainage tube over Amplatz guidewire and into abscess
- Advance metal stiffener up to abscess margin, but no further
- Will experience loss of resistance when tube passes into abscess
- Fix position of metal stiffener, and advance drainage tube into abscess
- Repeat CT images to confirm catheter is in correct location
- Consider irrigating abscess
- Sew catheter to skin or an adhesive device with 3-0 monofilament nylon
- Tape catheter securely with mesentery-style taping

Post-Procedure
Things to Do
- Record catheter output on graphics sheet q shift
- Flush catheter with 5-10 cc sterile, normal saline q 8 hours
- Follow catheter output, WBC (white blood cell count), fever and pain
- Persistent fever and leukocytosis after 1 to 2 days, often indicates undrained pus and a repeat CT scan should be obtained
- Signs of improvement include normalization of WBC count, afebrile, decreased drainage and resolution of abscess on CT scan

Common Problems & Complications
- Inadequate drainage due to loculated collection or fistula
- Abscesses unable to be drained percutaneously often require open surgery
- Bleeding
- Puncture of rectum
- Pain which may persist after catheter removal
- Catheter kink or dislodgement
- Bacteremia and septic shock
- Inadvertent dislodgement of tube
- Inadvertent dislodgement of metal ring from a dilator in thick ligaments

Selected References
1.   Ryan JM et al: Use of the transgluteal route for percutaneous abscess drainage in acute diverticulitis to facilitate delayed surgical repair [clinical conference]. AJR 170:1189-93, 1998
2.   Shah H et al: Saline injection into the perirectal space to assist transgluteal drainage of deep pelvic abscesses. JVIR 8:119-21, 1997
3.   Stallard DJ et al: Minor vascular anatomy of the abdomen and pelvis: A CT atlas. Radiographics 14:493-513, 1994

Transhepatic Cholangiogram

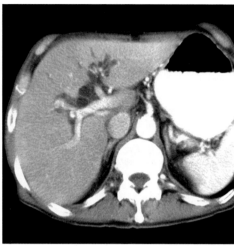

Important regions to check: 1) Which ducts are dilated, 2) Where is the site of obstruction, 3) Is left lobe of liver normal size or hypoplastic (affects whether can consider a left sided approach), 4) Location of large blood vessels relative to bile ducts, 5) Plan your approach.

Key Facts
- Synonyms: Percutaneous transhepatic cholangiogram (PTC)
- Initial attempts at biliary drainage are usually made with ERCP (endoscopic retrograde pancreatography) techniques
- Evaluation of an IV contrast enhanced CT scan is helpful for planning PTC

Pre-Procedure
Indications
- Most common indication is malignant biliary obstruction with unsuccessful attempt at ERCP
- Typically PTC is done as the initial part of a percutaneous biliary drainage (PBD) procedure such as placement of drainage catheters and stents
- Previous intestinal surgery which precludes ERCP
- Benign biliary obstruction with unsuccessful ERCP
- Evaluation of bile leak

Contraindications
- Uncorrectable bleeding diathesis
- Polycystic liver disease

Getting Started
- Things to Check
  - Bleeding history, platelets, PT, PTT, INR, creatinine and bilirubin
  - Check any prior CT scans, ERCPs (endoscopic retrograde cholangio-pancreatograms) or related studies
  - CT is very helpful for planning procedure
  - If procedure is elective, and a CT is not available, then obtain new CT
  - Check size and location of intrahepatic biliary ducts (IHDs) and relative position of portal vein branches
  - Check position of IHDs relative to T12 vertebra
  - Choose a peripheral bile duct to enter for PTC

Transhepatic Cholangiogram

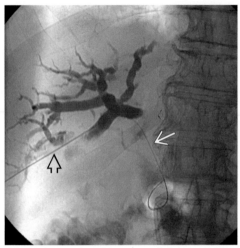

PTC from a right sided approach. A 21 gauge needle (open arrow) has been placed into a right sided duct and a 0.018" guidewire (white arrow) has been advanced into the CBD.

- o Seek a path which avoids large central blood vessels of liver to decrease risk of bleeding
- o Is liver herniated into chest with consequent increased risk of pleural space transgression and empyema or pneumothorax?
- o Check for colon anterior or lateral to liver
- o Look for a landmark that can be a guide to needle placement and is visible with fluoroscopy (fluoro) e.g. a radiopaque surgical clip
- o Check for tumors
- o Do not want to place a catheter through a tumor as may lead to excessive bleeding
- o Check size of left lobe of liver and for dilated IHDs in left lobe
  - ▪ If left lobe of liver is small, a left approach may be difficult
- • Equipment List
  - o Ultrasound if planning to do a left sided approach
  - o 21-gauge needle and 0.018" guidewire
  - o Coaxial dilator to upsize system from a 0.018" to 0.035" guidewire
  - o 40 cm long, 5 French hockey-stick-tip catheter

Prophylactic Antibiotics
- • Administer antibiotics to all patients
- • Relevant factors include patient's renal function and whether or not coverage for pseudomonas should be provided

Procedure

Patient Position
- • Supine
- • Prep skin from right posterior axillary line to left midclavicular line
- • Put CT scan hardcopy film on view box in procedure room

Procedure Steps
- • Obtain AP and RAO scout spot films
- • Can use right or left sided approach

Transhepatic Cholangiogram

- Right-sided approach is technically easier

<u>Right-Sided Approach</u>
- To help define lower extent of pleural space observe with fluoro as patient takes a deep breath
- 21 G needle placed over rib at lowest lateral intercostal space (e.g. just over 11th rib) in midaxillary line, and typically aimed towards T12 vertebra
  - Planned path of needle also depends on appearance of liver on CT and on fluoroscopy
  - Try to avoid large central vessels of liver
- Injection tubing is connected to needle hub
- Needle is slowly withdrawn in increments of a few millimeters and contrast is injected until a bile duct is opacified
- To minimize number of punctures of liver capsule, for additional needle passes, withdraw needle to liver margin without exiting liver
  - Then redirect needle path e.g. slightly more anterior or posterior
- Contrast can continue to be injected through needle to opacify bile ducts
  - Avoid overdistention of IHDs as may lead to bacteremia
- Alternatively, can use Seldinger technique to place a coaxial dilator, 0.035" guidewire and then 5 French hockey-stick-tip-catheter
- Obtain AP, RAO and LAO spot films

<u>Left-Sided Approach</u>
- Left IHDs are more anterior and contrast tends to quickly "wash out" as travels to more dependent common bile duct and left-sided ducts are also usually smaller than right
- If ascites is present, it is less likely to leak from an anterior left liver approach, than from a right midaxillary line entry site
- Ultrasound guidance is helpful for left approach

Post-Procedure
<u>Things to Do</u>
- Bed rest x 6 hours and continue antibiotics for at least 24 hours

Common Problems & Complications
- Pain
- Cholangitis and biliary sepsis
- Bleeding with perihepatic or intrahepatic hematoma or with hemobilia
- Pneumothorax and empyema
- Iodine contrast nephropathy

Selected References
1. Funaki B et al: Percutaneous biliary drainage in patients with nondilated intrahepatic bile ducts. AJR 173:1541-1544, 1999
2. Banerjee B et al: Percutaneous transcholecystic approach to the rendezvous procedure when transhepatic access fails. JVIR 5:895-8, 1994
3. Harbin WP et al: Transhepatic cholangiography: Complications and use patterns of the fine-needle technique: A multi-institutional survey. Radiology 135:15-22, 1980

Index of Procedures

NOTES

NOTES

NOTES

NOTES

NOTES

NOTES

NOTES

NOTES

NOTES

NOTES

NOTES

NOTES

NOTES

NOTES